Herbal Remedies

Discover the Healing Power of Medicinal Plants for a Healthy Life

Johanna Westwood

Table of Contents

Introduction

In modern world, where synthetic drugs often reign supreme, the idea of harnessing the power of nature might seem antiquated or simplistic. However, herbal remedies provide a wealth of benefits that can complement, and in some cases even offer alternatives to, conventional treatments.

Not for nothing in the recent decades, we've seen a resurgence in the interest surrounding herbal medicine. This revival stems from an increasingly felt need to return to nature, to seek holistic health practices, and to find sustainable, accessible alternatives to mainstream pharmaceuticals. While modern medicine undoubtedly has its strengths, it often lacks a holistic approach, and its focus on synthetic drugs leaves many people yearning for natural, time-tested solutions - which is precisely where herbal remedies come into play.

The power of herbal medicine is both subtle and profound. These remedies aren't just about addressing specific health issues. They're about promoting overall well-being, preventing disease, and cultivating a harmonious relationship between mind, body, and environment. They are about bringing us back into balance and enhancing our inherent healing capabilities.

We'll start this guide by delving into the rich history of herbal remedies, tracing their evolution from ancient times to our modern world. From there, we examine the philosophical foundations that underpin this form of healing, before moving on to the scientific principles that explain why and how these remedies work.

We'll then guide you through the different types of herbal medicines, helping you understand their unique characteristics, uses, and preparation methods. We'll also delve into a detailed discussion of various common ailments, from digestive and respiratory issues to cardiovascular and mental health conditions, and explore how herbal remedies can help manage and alleviate these health challenges.

You are part of a vibrant, interconnected web of life, and that your well-being is intrinsically linked to the health of this larger system.

So, with an open mind and a sense of curiosity, let's begin this healing and empowering journey together. Welcome to the incredible world of herbal remedies!

Chapter One: History and Principles

From time immemorial, humankind has turned to nature in the quest for healing. Illness presented a profound threat to survival, prompting a tireless search for remedies. It was observed that certain plants, when consumed or applied to wounds, could aid in combatting various afflictions. Thus, the narrative of herbal remedies was born.

Our understanding of these natural remedies has journeyed a considerable distance since those primordial times. The Babylonians, Egyptians, Chinese, and other ancient civilizations documented their knowledge of herbal remedies in medical texts. In China, "Shennong Ben Cao Jing" ("Shennong Emperor's Classic of Materia Medica"), penned during the Western Han dynasty (202 BC – 8 AD), stands as one of the earliest comprehensive studies of medicinal plants.

During the Middle Ages, when science and medicine in Europe were in their infancy, healers and monks meticulously preserved and disseminated the wisdom of plant-based healing. Works such as the "Great Herbal" (1485) cataloged hundreds of herbs and their therapeutic properties.

However, with the advent of the industrial era and the progression of pharmacology, interest in herbal remedies waned. Synthetic medicines became more accessible and predictable. Yet, this didn't signal the extinction of herbal remedies; they continued to be utilized in many cultures around the globe.

Today, as we stand at the dawn of the 21st century, we're witnessing a renaissance of herbal remedies. Physicians and researchers are increasingly acknowledging the value of these botanical aids, backed by centuries of experience and contemporary scientific investigation. Many individuals are consciously opting for more natural, environmentally friendly ways to maintain their health and well-being, where herbal remedies play a pivotal role.

This resurgence of herbal remedies doesn't represent a simple rejection of modern medicine. Rather, it testifies to our aspiration for integrative medicine, which marries traditional practices with modern scientific advancements. It showcases our desire for a balanced approach that harmonizes ancient wisdom with cutting-edge medical discoveries.

Principles

Beliefs and practices in herbalism exhibit a kaleidoscope of variations across the globe, yet they all share fundamental elements shaping the foundational philosophy of herbal remedies. These consist of viewing health as a holistic system, exhibiting reverence towards nature, and endorsing the individual's active participation in their healing journey.

In the holistic health model, the body is perceived as a complex system, where all parts are intricately interconnected, influencing one another. Consequently, an ailment or discomfort in one part of the body could signal more profound issues in another area. This model diverges from the traditional Western approach, which typically targets the alleviation of specific symptoms.

Herbal practitioners strive to understand and address the root causes of health issues, rather than merely focusing on symptom relief. They consider factors such as diet, lifestyle, stress, and emotional state, all of which can impact physical health.

Another vital aspect of the herbal remedy philosophy is respect for nature. Herbalists believe that nature provides everything necessary for our health and well-being. They value the diversity and complexity of the natural world, learning to explore and utilize these resources in a respectful and sustainable manner.

Herbalists also emphasize the importance of each individual actively participating in their healing process. This may involve learning and practicing the gathering and preparation of their own herbs, coupled with a deep understanding of how these impact the body. This approach empowers people to take greater control of their health and well-being. It also fosters self-awareness and self-respect, crucial elements of any healing journey.

It's essential to note that the philosophy of herbal remedies doesn't reject modern Western medicine. On the contrary, it aims to integrate with it, crafting a holistic approach to health and healing, utilizing the best aspects of both systems for optimal outcomes.

All these factors coalesce to form a unique and powerful philosophy underpinning the use of herbal remedies. They represent a fusion of our ancestors' wisdom and contemporary knowledge, urging a deeper understanding of our body and mind, and acknowledging the power of nature as a wellspring of health and well-being.

Each individual is bestowed with innate wisdom and the ability to care for their health. Through learning, practice, and experience, we all can become our own health experts, harnessing herbs to maintain and restore balance and well-being.

Herbal Remedies Today

In our era, the use of herbal remedies is experiencing a renaissance, becoming an increasingly active component of medical practices worldwide. Stemming from ancient traditions, herbalism continues to play a significant role in modern healthcare, profoundly influencing various facets of our lives.

Foremost, herbal remedies offer an alternative to contemporary pharmacology, often associated with a slew of side effects. They embody a more natural and holistic approach to health, aiming not only to alleviate symptoms but also eradicate the root causes of illnesses. As more and more people are seeking to incorporate natural methods into their lifestyle, herbal remedies are gaining increasing relevance.

Herbal remedies also play an essential role in providing accessible healthcare. Most herbs are readily available and economically priced, making them accessible to a broad populace, especially in developing countries where access to traditional medical aid may be limited.

The growing interest in herbal remedies helps preserve and propagate traditional medical knowledge. Much of this knowledge could be lost without the continual practice and study of herbal remedies. This process fosters respect and appreciation for cultural heritage and our planet's biological diversity.

Herbal remedies can also play a pivotal role in combating some of the most complex medical challenges of our time. For instance, they can propose novel approaches to managing chronic diseases such as diabetes and cardiovascular diseases, becoming increasingly prevalent in modern society.

Finally, herbal remedies play a critical role in mental health. Stress and anxiety are becoming more common in our rapidly changing world, and many individuals are turning to herbal remedies to restore balance and tranquility.

In the realm of scientific research, herbal remedies continue to prove their efficacy. Modern studies validate many claims made by ancient practices regarding the therapeutic properties of herbs, opening new horizons for developing innovative medicinal products and treatment strategies.

It's also worth noting that interest in self-care and preventative medicine is growing in today's society. Herbal remedies can offer a plethora of solutions in this context, helping individuals maintain their health and prevent diseases.

Know the Benefits, but do not Forget the Risks

Herbal remedies offer a wealth of benefits, making them a valuable addition to your health strategy. One of the most apparent advantages is their inherent naturalness. They embody a more holistic approach to health, one that considers your overall physical and emotional state, not merely disease symptoms.

Herbal remedies also provide a vast spectrum of treatment options. There's a herb or combination of herbs for almost any condition or symptom you're trying to alleviate, making them a versatile tool that can be tailored to your individual needs.

Additionally, herbal remedies are typically more accessible and cheaper than many modern medicines. Most herbs can be grown independently or purchased at an affordable price, making them an excellent choice for individuals with limited access to traditional medical aid or those who can't afford costly medications.

Furthermore, the use of herbal remedies can enhance your connection to the environment. Cultivating your medicinal herbs or gathering them in nature can help establish a deeper bond with the natural world and heighten your understanding of how it can support your health.

Lastly, herbal remedies promote self-sufficiency and management of personal health. They provide the tools for taking care of your health and making critical decisions concerning your well-being.

Since herbal remedies are natural and have been utilized for millennia, many people mistakenly consider them entirely safe. However, like any medicine, they carry risks that are crucial to understand for their effective and safe use. So, what about the risks?

One of the most common risks is the potential for allergic reactions. Some individuals might be allergic to specific herbs or their components. Moreover, some herbs may interact with medications you're already taking, causing unwanted side effects or diminishing the effectiveness of these drugs.

Some herbs can be toxic when exceeding recommended dosages, making it crucial always to adhere to dosage instructions. Additionally, certain herbs may be unsafe for specific groups of people, such as pregnant women, children, or individuals with certain chronic illnesses.

Chapter Two: Basics of Herbal Medicine

"Phytotherapy" is a term originated from Greek words - "phyto," meaning "plant," and "therapeia," which translates to "treatment." It is a globally recognized term used to refer to the medicinal application of plants.

It's essential to understand that herbal medicine is a diverse field, not a uniform one. It encompasses several types of herbal medicine, each with its unique philosophy, methodologies, and ways of using plants.

Western Herbal Medicine: This form of herbal medicine mainly targets specific symptoms using single herbs or herb mixtures. It is grounded in scientific research and clinical practice and often involves the study of plant pharmacology.

Traditional Chinese Medicine (TCM): This time-honored type of herbal medicine applies complex herb mixtures to bring balance to the body. It is centered around the notions of "qi" (life energy) and maintaining equilibrium between "yin" and "yang."

Ayurveda: This ancient Indian healthcare system uses herbs in combination with diet, yoga, and meditation to bring about a balance among body, mind, and spirit.

Naturopathy: This variant of herbal medicine focuses on holistic health and disease prevention. It utilizes various natural therapies, including herbal preparations, diet, exercise, and lifestyle modifications.

Despite their differing methodologies and philosophies, all these forms of herbal medicine acknowledge the fundamental role of nature in maintaining human health and promoting wellness.

Various forms of herbal preparations are used in these types of herbal medicine:

Dried Herbs: These are typically parts of plants, such as leaves, roots, flowers, seeds, bark, and stems, that are dried for preservation purposes. Often used to brew teas, decoctions, or infusions, dried herbs can extract potent components that offer medicinal benefits. They are also useful in cooking as spices or flavor enhancers. Some people choose to consume dried herbs in capsule or tablet form as dietary supplements.

Tinctures: This refers to concentrated liquid extracts created by immersing herbs in alcohol, which extracts the potent elements from the herbs. Although primarily taken internally, some tinctures can be used topically. They are effective in preserving the medicinal components of herbs over a long duration and are usually potent even in small amounts.

Extracts: These are products made by separating the active ingredients of herbs using various solvents such as water, alcohol, vinegar, glycerin, or oil. Available in both liquid and solid form, extracts are generally more potent than dried herbs or tinctures and often included in dietary supplements.

Ointments and creams: These are topical herbal formulations commonly used for treating a variety of skin conditions. Various bases like oil, wax, fat, or lanolin can be used to prepare ointments and creams. When applied directly to the skin, these preparations can effectively treat conditions such as eczema, psoriasis, burns, insect bites, among others.

Essential oils: These are highly concentrated liquids derived from plants using methods like steam distillation or cold pressing. Known to carry the distinctive aromatic and therapeutic properties, or the "essence," of the plant, essential oils are used widely in aromatherapy to evoke specific emotions or mental states. They can also be applied topically for skin ailments or inhaled for respiratory issues. However, due to their concentrated nature, essential oils should always be used cautiously, with dilution before applying to the skin, to prevent irritation or allergic reactions.

But what makes it tick? What makes some plants medicinal while others are not? To address these questions, we need to dive deep into the scientific principles that ground herbal medicine.

Plants create a multitude of substances, referred to as secondary metabolites. These are chemical compounds that serve a defensive purpose for plants against pests, diseases, and rival plant species. Many of these substances also hold beneficial attributes for human health. They can act as antioxidants, antibacterials, antivirals, anti-inflammatories, and other properties that are useful in battling various illnesses.

Scientific investigations in the realm of phytochemistry - the scientific branch dedicated to studying chemical compounds in plants - have shed light on how these substances interact with the human body. Here are some primary mechanisms via which herbal mixtures exert their influence:

Protein interactions: A multitude of herbal mixtures affect certain proteins in our bodies, altering their function. For instance, compounds from some plants may inhibit proteins responsible for inflammation, thus aiding in the reduction of inflammatory responses.

Enzyme regulation: Enzymes serve as the catalysts for chemical reactions in our bodies. Certain plant-based substances can either boost or restrict the activity of specific enzymes, thereby regulating biochemical processes.

Hormone influence: Some herbs can modulate hormone levels or imitate their actions, affecting various functions, from mood regulation to metabolic processes.

Direct microorganism combat: Some plants create substances that can directly eliminate bacteria, viruses, or fungi, making them effective in treating infections.

Antioxidant effects: Numerous plants contain antioxidants - substances that shield our cells from free radicals, unstable molecules that can harm cells and trigger chronic diseases.

Herbal medicine operates on diverse layers, imparting a comprehensive effect on the body. It's crucial to realize that each plant is comprised of hundreds of different substances that can interact with each other and with our bodies, yielding unique effects. This complexity makes herbal medicine a rich and intricate science, offering a vast landscape for exploration and utilization.

The science underpinning herbal medicine is an ever-evolving field. There is a growing body of research aimed at deciphering the workings of herbs, their efficacy, and safety parameters. This enables us to comprehend better how to tap into the power of plants to sustain health and promote well-being.

Distinguishing between Herbal and Conventional Medicine

Herbal and traditional medicine both strive to mitigate illnesses and foster health. However, their approaches, methodologies, and implications diverge significantly. In this chapter, we will delineate the primary distinctions between these two forms of medicine, while acknowledging that they can coexist in a well-rounded, integrative approach to health and wellness.

Philosophical Contrasts

The divergence between botanical and traditional medicine primarily stems from their foundational philosophies pertaining to health and illness.

Herbal Medicine: This typically adopts a holistic perspective, considering the body as a harmonized entity, and equating health with a balanced state within this system. Illness is often interpreted as a disruption of this equilibrium. Botanical medicine aims to reinstate this balance and enhance the body's inherent healing mechanisms.

Traditional Medicine: This often embraces a more compartmentalized viewpoint, perceiving the body as an assembly of distinct parts and systems. Illness is considered a malfunction within these elements and is typically addressed with treatments aimed at specific symptoms or disease pathways.

Methodologies and Therapies

Herbal Medicine: Therapeutic strategies typically involve extracts from whole plants consisting of a variety of active compounds. These treatments usually exert a gentle, systemic influence, helping to reestablish the body's overall balance and boost its natural healing responses. Botanical practitioners often tailor treatments to the individual's comprehensive health, lifestyle, and personal circumstances.

Traditional Medicine: Therapeutic strategies typically entail synthetic drugs that target specific biological pathways. These drugs usually deliver faster, more pronounced results, with their dosages and impacts being generally predictable and standardized.

Research and Oversight

Herbal Medicine: Research into botanical medicine has been less extensive, primarily due to funding constraints. Despite many herbs having been safely used for centuries with substantial anecdotal backing, fewer have undergone stringent scientific trials. Botanical remedies are also less regulated, leading to potential issues in quality control.

Traditional Medicine: These treatments undergo thorough research and stringent testing prior to approval. They are also strictly regulated, ensuring consistent quality and safety.

Accessibility and Pricing

Herbal Medicine: Botanical remedies tend to be more accessible and cost-effective, particularly in regions where contemporary healthcare services are scarce or costly. Many herbs can be homegrown or collected from the wild.

Traditional Medicine: Traditional treatments can be costly and less accessible, especially in less-developed countries. However, they are often covered by health insurance policies, which is typically not the case for botanical remedies.

While botanical and traditional medicine vary considerably, they can be regarded as complementary rather than rivaling approaches. Many health practitioners now advocate for an integrative approach, acknowledging that both forms of medicine have their strengths and shortcomings, and can collaborate to deliver optimal care for patients.

Legal and Ethical Aspects

While botanical medicine boasts a rich historical lineage, the legality and ethical implications of its application are intricate and perpetually in flux. These implications span from quality assurance and product regulation to intellectual property and sustainability. This chapter will explore various legal and ethical dimensions of botanical medicine.

Regulation and Quality Assurance

The regulatory landscape of botanical products differs significantly across countries. In some regions, they are considered dietary supplements and, as such, are not subjected to the same intensive testing and quality assurance as traditional drugs. This can result in quality inconsistencies, with some products lacking the specified ingredients in the stated quantities, or being tainted with additional substances. For consumers, this highlights the necessity of opting for products from trustworthy sources and manufacturers.

Safety and Efficiency

In numerous jurisdictions, botanical remedies, by virtue of being categorized as dietary supplements, are not obliged to establish safety and efficiency prior to market entry. While many herbs have a well-established history of traditional application and some scientific backing for their benefits, others are yet to be extensively examined. Additionally, the possibility of side effects, allergic reactions, and interactions with other medication implies that botanical remedies should be used judiciously.

Intellectual Property Rights

Intellectual property rights present a notable ethical challenge in the realm of botanical medicine. Many medicinal plants have been harnessed by indigenous communities over centuries, with their traditional knowledge significantly enriching the global pharmacopoeia. However, when pharmaceutical corporations patent plant compounds for their utilization, it may incite issues of biopiracy and exploitation. Respecting and recognizing the rights of indigenous communities is imperative in this regard.

Sustainability

Rising demand for botanical products can strain wild plant populations, resulting in overharvesting and endangering biodiversity. Ethical botanical remedy providers are obligated to procure their ingredients in a sustainable manner, safeguarding the environment and the communities that rely on these plants. Consumers can contribute to this by choosing products from firms that emphasize sustainable sourcing and fair trade practices.

Professional Conduct

For those practicing botanical medicine, legal and ethical standards must be upheld. These include securing informed consent from patients, respecting patient confidentiality, and perpetually aiming to uphold superior standards of care. Practitioners ought to possess appropriate training and qualifications and stay abreast of the latest developments in their field.

Chapter Three: Herbs and Their Properties

In the field of plant-based healing, various categories exist to classify herbs. This is determined by their healing properties, the influence they have on the human organism, their botanical lineage, among other criteria. This chapter uncovers several common strategies of herb classification in plant-based healing, a comprehension that can help novices better understand and steer through the broad realm of plant-based remedies.

Classification Driven by Healing Applications

Often, herbs are grouped according to their healing properties or the health issues and symptoms they can counteract. For example:

Adaptogens: Adaptogens are a distinctive group of herbs that aid the body in adjusting to both physical and mental stress factors. Their role centers around bolstering the adrenal glands, pivotal organs in the body's response to stress. They not only help stabilize hormone levels but also reinforce overall health by fortifying immunity and encouraging quality sleep. Ginseng, for instance, is valued for its energy-enhancing properties and its ability to boost mental sharpness. Ashwagandha, another famed adaptogen, has been observed to lower cortisol levels, mitigate stress and anxiety, and foster improved sleep. Rhodiola is often used for its capacity to counteract fatigue and depression, elevate work productivity, and reduce signs of stress-induced exhaustion.

Analgesics: These herbs are traditionally harnessed for pain relief. For example, willow bark has been a remedy for pain and inflammation for countless generations. It contains a chemical known as salicin, which transforms into salicylic acid in the body — the precursor to aspirin. Turmeric is another potent analgesic owing to its active element, curcumin, which is recognized for its potent anti-inflammatory and antioxidant properties. These herbs are frequently used in addressing conditions like arthritis, muscle pain, and headaches.

Antimicrobials: These herbs have properties that battle bacteria, viruses, or fungi. Garlic, for instance, contains a compound named allicin which is a strong antimicrobial agent, believed to be effective against a broad variety of bacteria and fungi. Echinacea has traditionally been harnessed to counter infections and fortify the immune system. It's commonly used in the treatment of colds and flu. Goldenseal also boasts antimicrobial properties and is usually harnessed to address digestive and respiratory infections.

Carminatives: These herbs are beneficial for the digestive system and aid in relieving digestive discomforts such as gas, bloating, and stomach cramps. Peppermint has a calming effect on the gastrointestinal tract, which can help soothe conditions like irritable bowel syndrome. Fennel has been a remedy for digestive issues, including heartburn, bloating, and loss of appetite, for countless generations. Chamomile is also well-recognized for its soothing properties, making it a frequent remedy for problems like indigestion, nausea, and gas.

Hypotensives: These herbs aid in regulating blood pressure levels. Hawthorn is traditionally used for heart health, with studies indicating that it can help reduce high blood pressure and protect against heart disease. Garlic, besides being an antimicrobial, has been discovered to provide significant cardiovascular benefits, including blood pressure reduction. Celery seed is also renowned for its hypotensive properties. It's frequently used to manage hypertension, but also has diuretic properties, which can further assist in lowering blood pressure by lessening the body's fluid content.

Classification Based on Effects on the Body Systems

Herbs are also sorted based on the physiological systems they mainly target:

Cardiovascular herbs: These are the herbs that significantly impact the heart and blood vessels, whether by fortifying the heart muscle, encouraging blood flow, or moderating blood pressure. Hawthorn, for instance, is hailed for its heart-shielding attributes and is applied to manage conditions like congestive heart failure, erratic heartbeats, and hypertension. Garlic has a remarkable influence in reducing blood pressure and cholesterol, thus fostering overall heart health. Motherwort is utilized to aid with heart ailments, including heart failure, irregular heartbeats, and heart symptoms associated with anxiety. It is thought to help alleviate heart palpitations and regulate an accelerated heartbeat.

Digestive herbs: These herbs can bolster the digestive system by promoting digestion, reducing inflammation in the stomach and intestines, and assisting in mitigating conditions such as bloating, indigestion, and nausea. Ginger is a formidable digestive herb, renowned for mitigating symptoms like nausea, vomiting, and indigestion. Peppermint offers solace to the gastrointestinal tract and aids with symptoms like bloating and gas. Milk thistle is primarily engaged to fortify the liver, but it also stimulates digestion and can aid in relieving constipation.

Nervous system herbs: These herbs engage with the brain and nerves, generally by soothing the nervous system, lessening anxiety, or facilitating sleep. Lemon balm is celebrated for its calming properties and is regularly used to lessen stress and anxiety, enhance sleep, and mitigate symptoms of indigestion. Lavender also has potent calming properties and is routinely used to alleviate anxiety, stress, and insomnia. Passionflower is commonly used for its sedative and sleep-inducing properties, making it beneficial for those grappling with insomnia or anxiety.

Respiratory herbs: These herbs bolster the lungs and airways, typically by mitigating inflammation, loosening mucus, or acting as an expectorant. Mullein is traditionally employed for respiratory issues, including chronic bronchitis, asthma, and tuberculosis. Eucalyptus is recognized for its capacity to help clear mucus from the lungs and enhance breathing. Elderberry has immune-fortifying properties and is often used to manage respiratory infections like the flu and common cold.

Urinary herbs: These herbs influence the kidneys and bladder, typically by fostering urination, aiding in the expulsion of toxins, or combating urinary tract infections. Dandelion leaf functions as a diuretic, augmenting urine production to help the body expel excess fluid. Cranberry is predominantly known for its role in warding off urinary tract infections by hindering bacteria from adhering to the urinary tract. Uva ursi is often used for urinary tract disorders, including infections of the kidney, bladder, and urethra, and it's praised for its robust antibacterial attributes.

Moreover, herbs can be sorted by their botanical families, as plants within identical families frequently exhibit similar characteristics and utilities. Some prevalent botanical families in herbal therapy encompass:

Lamiaceae (mint family): Also referred to as the mint or deadnettle family, this clan encompasses roughly 236 genera and over 7,000 species. A substantial number of these bear a strong aroma due to the essential oils found within the plants. Members of this family are often utilized in culinary practices for flavoring, in the creation of perfumes, and in both conventional and contemporary medicine. For instance, peppermint is extensively employed for its cooling and calming influences, particularly when managing digestive complications like irritable bowel syndrome. Sage, notable for its antimicrobial properties, is often used for oral health, while also being hailed for its potential cognition-enhancing effects. Rosemary, besides being a popular culinary herb, has been used for its potential to bolster digestion, circulation, and neurological health, including memory enhancement.

Asteraceae (daisy family): Also referred to as the aster, daisy, or sunflower family, this is the largest family of vascular plants with over 23,000 species. Echinacea, a prominent member of this family, is acclaimed for its immune-fortifying properties and is frequently used to prevent and manage common colds and other infections. Dandelion, sometimes dismissed as a weed, is abundant in vitamins and minerals, and both its leaves and root have been used for liver detoxification, as a digestive aid, and for skin conditions. Chamomile, a herb lauded for its calming attributes, is often consumed as a tea to foster relaxation and assist sleep, but also has an extensive history of use for conditions like digestive ailments and skin issues.

Apiaceae (carrot family): Also known as the parsley or celery family, the Apiaceae family includes about 3,700 species. It encompasses several herbs known for their medicinal and culinary applications. Caraway seeds are recognized for their carminative properties and are often used to mitigate symptoms of indigestion including bloating and gas. Fennel, which is both a culinary herb and a medicinal plant, is frequently used to manage digestive issues and can also function as a diuretic. Angelica, a potent medicinal herb within this family, is used for various purposes including digestive disorders and coughs.

Its root is acclaimed for its warming and stimulating impact on circulation, and it's also used to flavor liqueurs and confectionery.

Common Herbs and Their Medicinal Uses

An array of plants hold value in herbal medicine, each with its distinctive qualities. This passage aims to introduce you to some typically found herbs, be it as part of your garden landscape, culinary ingredients, or therapeutic aids.

Peppermint (Mentha piperita): Peppermint, a fusion of spearmint and watermint, is native to Europe and the Middle East. The refreshing aroma it's renowned for stems from its active substance, menthol, which also contributes to its numerous medicinal effects. As a carminative, peppermint pacifies the smooth muscles of the gastrointestinal tract, providing relief from discomforts such as bloating, gas, and indigestion. Its antispasmodic attributes make it useful for ailments such as irritable bowel syndrome (IBS). Additionally, peppermint oil harbors antimicrobial properties and can be topically applied for easing muscle and joint pain. Recent studies also hint that it could aid in boosting memory and cognitive functioning.

Chamomile (Matricaria recutita): Chamomile, praised for its gentle, soothing attributes, has been employed in herbal medicine for centuries. Its flowers, rich in essential oils and other advantageous compounds, are customarily brewed into a calming tea. Chamomile imparts a calming effect on the nervous system, making it a favored option for lessening stress and anxiety, and encouraging restful sleep.

It also has anti-inflammatory properties which can assist in soothing gastrointestinal troubles like indigestion, gastritis, and ulcerative conditions. When used topically, chamomile can help decrease inflammation and expedite skin healing, proving useful for conditions like eczema, wounds, or burns.

Echinacea (Echinacea spp.): Echinacea, also known as the purple coneflower, is a group of flowering plants indigenous to North America. It's highly esteemed in traditional medicine for its immunity-boosting properties. Echinacea is thought to bolster the immune system by stimulating the activation of white blood cells, our body's primary defense against pathogens. This makes it especially useful for preventing and treating colds, flu, and other respiratory infections. Some research also suggests that echinacea might showcase anti-inflammatory and antioxidant properties, and could potentially aid in managing skin disorders and wound healing.

Lavender (Lavandula spp.): Lavender is a group of 47 recognized species of flowering plants in the mint family, originating from the Old World. It's recognized for its distinctive aroma, purple-blue flowers, and wide usage in aromatherapy, perfumery, and culinary endeavors. Its essential oil, derived from the flowers, carries its medicinal value. Lavender is celebrated for its calming and relaxing properties and is often used to address conditions like anxiety, stress, and insomnia. It can be used in several forms, including teas, tinctures, and essential oils for diffusion or topical application. Lavender also has antimicrobial properties, making it beneficial for topical application on minor wounds, burns, and specific skin conditions.

Turmeric (Curcuma longa): This plant is part of the ginger family and easily recognized by its vibrant yellow-orange hue, playing a crucial role as a spice in numerous Asian dishes. Its active ingredient, curcumin, possesses anti-inflammatory and antioxidant capabilities. These attributes render turmeric an often-resorted-to solution for inflammation and joint pain, such as those found in arthritis. Emerging studies also hint that curcumin might enhance endothelial function, thus benefiting heart health, and might present advantages for brain health, inclusive of potential protective effects against neurodegenerative disorders like Alzheimer's disease.

Ginger (Zingiber officinale): Known as a blooming plant, ginger's rhizome, or underground stem, is widely used as a spice and in traditional medicine. It originates from Southeast Asia and shares a close kinship with turmeric. In the medical realm, ginger is most renowned for its ability to alleviate digestive disturbances, especially nausea and vomiting related to motion sickness, pregnancy, and chemotherapy. Additionally, it contains compounds known as gingerols and shogaols, which possess anti-inflammatory and antioxidant properties. These qualities render ginger beneficial for managing inflammatory conditions like arthritis and can bolster overall immune health. Upcoming research also suggests potential benefits for cardiovascular health, such as reducing blood pressure and cholesterol levels.

Milk Thistle (Silybum marianum): Also referred to as Saint Mary's thistle, Milk thistle is an herbaceous plant hailing from the Asteraceae family. Although native to the Mediterranean region, it is now found globally. The plant's distinct features include its purple flower and white-veined leaves. The active ingredient in milk thistle, silymarin, is primarily found in the seeds and is a group of flavonoids. Known as a potent antioxidant and anti-inflammatory compound, silymarin has been widely used in traditional medicine to aid liver health. It is believed to safeguard liver cells from damage by preventing the entry of harmful toxins and aiding in the elimination of these toxins from liver cells. Additionally, silymarin has demonstrated an ability to promote liver cell regeneration, offering a therapeutic effect for liver-related disorders such as cirrhosis, jaundice, hepatitis, and gallbladder diseases.

Ginkgo (Ginkgo biloba): More commonly referred to as just ginkgo or the maidenhair tree, Ginkgo biloba is among the most ancient living tree species on Earth. Native to China, ginkgo trees have been cultivated for millennia for their varied medicinal benefits. Ginkgo leaves are packed with flavonoids and terpenoids, compounds celebrated for their potent antioxidant effects. These compounds are believed to enhance blood circulation, particularly to the brain, and protect nerve cells from damage, thus potentially improving cognitive function and memory. As a result, it has gained popularity in treating cognitive impairments, such as dementia, Alzheimer's disease, and concentration issues. Some research also suggests that ginkgo might help with conditions like tinnitus, vertigo, and certain eye problems like macular degeneration.

St. John's Wort (Hypericum perforatum): St. John's Wort, a flower-bearing plant, thrives in the wild across Europe and has spread to other temperate zones around the globe. The name 'St. John's Wort' stems from its traditional blossoming and harvesting period around St. John's Day, June 24. The plant, distinguished by its radiant yellow flowers, contains several active ingredients, including hypericin and hyperforin. These ingredients are believed to influence specific neurotransmitters, helping elevate and stabilize mood. Consequently, St. John's Wort is commonly used to manage mild to moderate depression, anxiety, and sleep disorders. Nonetheless, it's crucial to recognize that St. John's Wort can interact with a variety of medications, encompassing antidepressants, contraceptives, and blood thinners. Therefore, prior to starting a St. John's Wort regimen, especially if other medications are involved, consulting with a healthcare provider is essential.

Elderberry (Sambucus nigra): Elderberry, a category of blooming plants within the Adoxaceae family, originates from most parts of Europe, northwest Africa, and western Asia. Its dark purple berries are packed with anthocyanins, offering powerful antioxidant and anti-inflammatory properties. Elderberries have been praised for their immune-strengthening benefits and used over centuries to combat colds and flu. They can be enjoyed in various forms, including syrups, teas, and capsules. Besides enhancing immune function, some studies suggest that elderberry may support cardiovascular health, promote healthy aging, and potentially assist with diabetes management.

Rosemary (Rosmarinus officinalis): Rosemary, a fragrant perennial herb, is native to the Mediterranean. Although it's widely acknowledged as a culinary herb, it also boasts an extensive history of medicinal application. Rosemary's active ingredients encompass rosmarinic acid, camphor, and caffeic acid, which account for its therapeutic properties. Traditionally, it's employed to bolster digestion and alleviate muscle and joint pain linked to inflammation. Its carnosic acid and rosmarinic acid components could enhance memory and focus and shield the brain against neurodegenerative diseases such as Alzheimer's. Some studies also suggest rosemary's potential in mood enhancement, immunity boosting, and liver health support.

Garlic (Allium sativum): Garlic, a species belonging to the onion genus, Allium, is indigenous to Central Asia and northeastern Iran. Celebrated for its distinctive taste, it's a staple ingredient in cuisines globally. The healthful attributes of garlic primarily come from its sulfur compounds, like allicin, which emerge when garlic cloves are cut or crushed. Traditionally, garlic has been used for cardiovascular wellness due to its ability to lower blood pressure and cholesterol levels. It also boasts formidable antimicrobial properties, making it effective against a variety of bacterial, viral, and fungal infections. Some studies suggest garlic might have potential anticancer properties.

Aloe Vera (Aloe barbadensis miller): Aloe Vera belongs to the succulent plant species within the Aloe genus, with its roots in the Arabian Peninsula. The dense, juicy leaves of this plant encase a gel brimming with vitamins, minerals, and a multitude of bioactive components. This gel has been applied externally for millennia to alleviate various skin issues. Given its soothing, anti-inflammatory, and wound-healing abilities, Aloe Vera is often the go-to for burns, lacerations, skin rashes, and sunburn. It can also address conditions like psoriasis and cold sores. Some people also ingest aloe vera juice for digestive troubles, but it's essential to proceed with care as it can induce laxative effects.

Hawthorn (Crataegus spp.): Hawthorn refers to a genus of bushes and trees in the Rosaceae family, native to the temperate zones of the Northern Hemisphere. It's a crucial element in herbal medicine for maintaining heart health. The berries, leaves, and flowers of Hawthorn are enriched with flavonoids and other compounds known for their antioxidant and anti-inflammatory properties. Hawthorn is reputed for its positive impact on heart function, potentially through enhanced blood vessel dilation, improved blood flow to the heart, and amplified heart muscle contractions. It's employed to manage heart failure symptoms and circulatory system-related conditions, such as hypertension and angina.

Dandelion (Taraxacum officinale): The dandelion is a widespread meadow herb within the Asteraceae family, originating from Eurasia, but now it's found in many regions worldwide. Often dismissed as a mere weed, the dandelion is in fact a nutritional powerhouse, offering a rich source of vitamins A, C, and K, along with minerals like iron, potassium, and zinc. Its leaves are recognized for their diuretic properties, proving beneficial in detoxifying the kidneys and urinary tract. The root is frequently used as a liver tonic, believed to prompt bile production and enhance digestion. The flowers have found their use in topical solutions for skin health. The entire plant is edible and can be incorporated into salads, brewed as tea, or used as a coffee alternative.

Chapter Four: Preparing Herbal Remedies

Crafting your plant-based remedies is a significant part of herbal medicine. The method of preparation often depends on the herb in question and its purpose, as certain techniques can enhance the medicinal potential of the plant. In this section, we'll explore a few commonly used preparation techniques, such as brewing teas, creating tinctures, formulating salves, and more.

Teas (Infusions and Decoctions): Herbal teas, often referred to as infusions or decoctions, represent a straightforward and prevalent approach to using medicinal plants.

Infusions are usually preferred for softer plant components like leaves, flowers, and seeds. To craft an infusion, pour boiling water over the chosen herbs and allow them to seep for 10-15 minutes before straining.

Decoctions, on the other hand, are used for tougher plant materials, such as roots, barks, and berries. These parts require a more rigorous extraction process. To create a decoction, simmer the herbs in water for 15-30 minutes before straining.

Consumed as beverages, these teas deliver medicinal benefits and can also be applied topically to address skin conditions.

Tinctures: Tinctures are a widely embraced means of preparing and administering herbal remedies. They're essentially concentrated herbal extracts, achieved by soaking (macerating) plant components in a solvent (such as alcohol or vinegar) over several weeks. This approach draws out the active compounds from the herbs, resulting in a highly potent liquid that can be administered in small quantities, usually dropped under the tongue (sublingually) or diluted in water. The alcohol base also serves as a preservative, maintaining the tincture's potency and efficacy for several years. Tinctures are particularly handy when rapid absorption is needed or when dealing with herbs that might be unpleasant in other forms.

Salves and Ointments: Salves and ointments are typically used for topical applications. They're made by infusing herbal components into a fatty base like oil or beeswax. This base is then usually blended with more beeswax or another thickening agent to produce a semi-solid substance that can be applied to the skin. Salves and ointments can transfer the therapeutic properties of the herbs directly to skin issues like wounds, burns, rashes, or dry or irritated skin. They're also commonly appreciated for their soothing, moisturizing, and protective features.

Capsules: Herbal capsules consist of powdered herbs encased in small, digestible shells. They offer a handy method of taking herbal medicine, especially for those who may find some herbs' flavor unpalatable in tea or tincture forms. Capsules deliver a consistent and precise dosage, and they're portable for travel or on-the-go use. However, it's crucial to remember that due to the processing involved, capsules might not offer the same potency as freshly prepared herbal teas or tinctures. Also, not all herbs are suitable for encapsulation, particularly those that are most effective when consumed fresh or as liquid extracts.

Syrups: Herbal syrups represent a favored method of ingesting medicinal plants, especially for those who may be deterred by the natural flavor of certain herbs. The process of creating an herbal syrup usually involves preparing a potent herbal tea or decoction and incorporating sweetening agents such as honey or sugar. These sweeteners not only enhance the taste of the medicinal mixture but also serve as natural preservatives, extending the syrup's shelf life. Syrups are versatile and can be used to treat various conditions, though they're particularly prevalent in remedies for respiratory concerns like coughs and sore throats, as they can alleviate throat irritation. Herbal syrups are also perfect for children who might find other forms of herbal medicine too potent or bitter to their taste.

Poultices and Compresses: Poultices and compresses are two forms of topical herbal applications that are remarkably effective for skin ailments, injuries, inflammation, and discomfort. A poultice is prepared by crushing herbs into a paste (or rehydrating dried herbs with a touch of hot water) and applying this concoction directly to the problem area. The herb-laden paste is generally enveloped in a piece of sterile cloth and left on the skin for several hours. Conversely, a compress is created by immersing a piece of cloth in an herbal infusion or decoction and then placing this soaked cloth onto the affected area. Both techniques enable the beneficial properties of the herbs to permeate directly through the skin and into the underlying tissues. Depending on the situation, a poultice or compress might be applied hot (to relax muscles or draw out infections) or cold (to minimize inflammation).

Preparing Herbal Teas and Decoctions

Enjoying the health benefits of medicinal plants through herbal teas and decoctions is straightforward and common. Let's take a detailed journey on how to concoct these at home.

Herbal Teas (Infusions)

Herb Selection: Determine the herbs you want to incorporate in your infusion. This could be a solitary herb or a mixture, depending on the effects you aim for.

Herb Quantification: The standard ratio usually stands at 1 tablespoon of dried herb or 2 tablespoons of fresh herb for every cup of water. However, this may change depending on the herb in question and your personal taste.

Water Boiling: Heat a pot of water until it boils.

Water Pouring: Deposit your herbs in a teapot or jar and pour the boiling water on top of them.

Steeping: Cap the container and allow your herbs to steep for roughly 10-15 minutes. You can modify this duration based on the intensity you prefer.

Straining and Consumption: Filter the infusion into a cup, discarding the used herbs. You can sweeten the tea with honey or other natural sweeteners if you wish.

Herbal Decoctions

Herb Selection: Pick the tough parts of herbs such as roots, barks, or berries for your decoction.

Herb Quantification: This step mirrors that of tea preparation.

Mixing Herbs and Water: Deposit your herbs into a pot and douse them with water.

Simmering: Elevate the water to boiling point, then lower the heat and allow the concoction to simmer. The hard plant materials necessitate a longer duration to divulge their medicinal virtues, hence it should simmer for 15-30 minutes.

Straining and Consumption: Post-simmering, strain the decoction into a cup, discarding the used herbs. If you wish, the decoction can be sweetened.

It's vital to remember that the boiling water may obliterate some properties of herbs, and therefore, not all herbs are apt for teas and decoctions. Always conduct comprehensive research on individual herbs to ensure you're utilizing the most suitable preparation technique.

Making Your Own Herbal Tinctures and Infusions

Crafting personal herbal tinctures and infusions is a pragmatic and fulfilling approach to tap into the potential of medicinal plants. These concoctions can serve various purposes for health and wellness.

Tinctures

Select Your Herb: The initial move in crafting a tincture is deciding on the herb or mix of herbs to use. This will hinge on the specific health advantages you're seeking. Fresh herbs are usually the preferred choice for tinctures as they can yield a richer flavor and potent medicinal attributes. Nevertheless, premium dried herbs can also create efficient tinctures. Remember to look up your selected herb for any potential adverse effects or contradictions, especially if you're on other medication or have prevailing health issues.

Process Your Herbs: Fresh herbs need to be thoroughly cleaned to eliminate any dirt or impurities. Post-cleaning, the herbs need to be finely sliced or crushed to amplify the surface area, which aids in extracting more beneficial compounds during the steeping phase. If using dried herbs, they're typically ready to use, although larger pieces may require crushing or grinding.

Quantify Your Herbs and Alcohol: Achieving the right herb-to-alcohol ratio is crucial for a potent tincture. For fresh herbs, a standard ratio is 1 part herb to 5 parts alcohol (1:5). Dried herbs, being more concentrated, follow a 1 part herb to 4 parts alcohol ratio (1:4). For instance, if you're using 100 grams of fresh herbs, you'd need 500 milliliters of alcohol.

Merge the Herbs and Alcohol: The herbs need to be deposited in a clean, dry glass jar. The alcohol is then poured over the herbs, completely immersing them. The alcohol acts as a solvent, extracting the medicinal constituents from the plant material.

Seal and Preserve: Once merged, the jar needs to be firmly sealed to prevent the alcohol from evaporating. The jar should be kept in a cool, dark place, like a pantry or cupboard, shielded from direct sunlight, which can deteriorate the herbs over time.

Agitate Regularly: The jar needs to be shaken daily. This ensures the alcohol can access all parts of the herbs and effectively extract the medicinal components.

Filter: The tincture should be ready to strain between 4 to 6 weeks. A fine-mesh strainer or cheesecloth can be utilized to separate the solid herb material from the liquid. Squeezing or pressing the herbs will extract as much liquid as possible.

Bottle and Identify: The completed tincture should be transferred into dark glass bottles to protect it from light degradation. Bottles with a dropper facilitate easy administration of the tincture. Each bottle needs to be labeled with the herb's name, the bottling date, and the used herb-to-alcohol ratio. This will assist you in keeping track, especially if you have multiple tinctures.

Making Herbal Infusions

Select Your Herb: Initiate by determining which herb or blend of herbs you aim to introduce into the oil. The selection will rely on your intended usage for the oil. Skin care frequently employs herbs like calendula, lavender, and chamomile, while for culinary infusions one might lean towards rosemary, thyme, or basil. Both fresh and dried herbs can be utilized. If using fresh herbs, ensure they are washed and fully dried to prevent water from getting into the oil, which could lead to rancidity.

Quantify Your Herbs and Oil: The proportion of herbs and oil can slightly vary, but a common rule of thumb is to fill your jar around half to three-quarters with herbs. Then, fill up the jar with oil until the herbs are completely submerged, to ensure full extraction of the medicinal properties of the herbs into the oil.

Merge the Herbs and Oil: Having measured your herbs and oil, place the herbs in your jar and pour the oil on top. Stir the mixture with a clean spoon or chopstick to eliminate any trapped air bubbles and confirm all herb material is in contact with the oil.

Seal and Preserve: After combining your herbs and oil, securely seal the jar. Then, locate the jar in a warm, sunlit spot, like a windowsill. The warmth and light will facilitate the extraction process, drawing the beneficial compounds from the herbs into the oil over a span of about 4 to 6 weeks.

Filter: Post-infusion period, filter the oil through a fine-mesh strainer or cheesecloth to separate the herbs from the oil. Make sure to squeeze or press the herb material to extract as much oil as feasible.

Bottle and Identify: Pour the filtered oil into a clean jar or bottle for storage. Don't forget to label your jar with the names of the used herbs and the date of the infusion. This assists in remembering the contents and creation date of each jar, especially if you make multiple infusions. Keep the oil in a cool, dark location to maintain its potency and prolong its shelf life.

Make sure to keep your tinctures and infusions in a cool, dark location and consume them within a year. As with any herbal remedy, it is advised to consult with a healthcare provider or professional herbalist prior to usage, particularly if you're pregnant, nursing, have any health conditions, or are on any other medication.

Crafting Herbal Salves, Ointments, and Lotions

Creating topical herbal concoctions like salves, ointments, and lotions can be a fulfilling process. Each of these carries distinct textures and uses.

Making Herbal Salves and Ointments

1. Select Your Herbs: The initial step involves choosing the herbs to incorporate in your salve or ointment. The selection depends on the specific attributes you want your salve to possess. For instance, if the objective is skin

healing, you might opt for herbs like calendula (known for its anti-inflammatory and antimicrobial characteristics), plantain (soothing and promotes healing), or comfrey (famed for its wound healing and skin irritation soothing properties).

Craft an Herbal Infused Oil: Having decided on your herbs, the following step is to imbue them into a carrier oil. This process entails placing the herbs in a jar, immersing them in oil, and allowing the mix to steep for several weeks. This duration allows the medicinal attributes of the herbs to seep into the oil. Ideal choices for carrier oils include olive oil, sweet almond oil, and coconut oil, given their skin-nourishing properties.

Sieve the Infused Oil: Post-infusion, filter the herbs from the oil using a fine-mesh strainer or cheesecloth. Be sure to press or squeeze the herbs to extract maximum oil.

Introduce Beeswax: The subsequent step involves adding beeswax to the infused oil. Beeswax's role is to solidify the oil, transforming it into a salve or ointment. For a stiffer salve, a typical proportion is about one part beeswax to four parts infused oil. For a softer ointment, incorporate less beeswax. Melt the beeswax in a double boiler, then blend it with the infused oil, stirring until the mixture is homogeneous.

Transfer to Containers: When the beeswax and oil have thoroughly mixed, pour the liquid blend into small, clean jars or tins.

Allow Cooling: Let the blend cool entirely. Upon cooling, the beeswax solidifies, morphing the blend into a solid salve or ointment.

Cover and Tag: Once the salve has entirely cooled and solidified, put lids on the jars or tins and tag them with the date, the type of salve or ointment, and the used herbs. This procedure helps you remember the purpose of each salve and its production date. Store the salve in a cool, dark spot when not in active use.

Making Herbal Lotions

Craft an Herbal Infused Oil: The inception of creating an herbal lotion involves crafting an herbal imbued oil. This encompasses steeping your selected herbs in a carrier oil (like olive oil, almond oil, or grapeseed oil) over several weeks, then filtering the herbs. The resultant oil retains the therapeutic properties of the herbs.

Assemble a Water Phase: The water aspect of your lotion can comprise distilled water, a floral hydrosol, aloe vera juice, or any other water-based fluid that aligns with your herb choice. For instance, for a rosemary lotion, you might opt for rosemary hydrosol. The quantity of your water phase should be approximately equal to that of your oil phase.

Develop an Emulsion: To blend the water phase and oil phase (which naturally tend to separate), you need to develop an emulsion. This requires heating the two phases in distinct double boilers until they reach an identical temperature, then gradually introducing the water phase into the oil phase while stirring persistently. The outcome is a homogeneous blend of oil and water.

Integrate a Natural Emulsifier: To ensure the oil and water remain blended, incorporate a natural emulsifier such as beeswax, lecithin, or borax. These should be melted into the oil phase prior to introducing the water phase.

Cool and Include Preservatives: Post formation of the emulsion, let it cool. If you wish to prolong your lotion's shelf life, you can integrate a natural preservative like grapefruit seed extract, vitamin E oil, or rosemary antioxidant extract at this stage. These help inhibit bacterial and mold growth.

Pour into Containers and Label: Once the lotion has cooled and thickened, transfer it into clean vessels and tag them with the lotion's name, the production date, and the utilized ingredients. Store your lotion in a cool, dark location when not in active use. It's generally advisable to use homemade lotions within a few months, especially if they lack preservatives.

Chapter Five: Digestive Disorders

Digestive complications encompass an extensive variety of ailments impacting the components of the gastrointestinal (GI) tract, which includes the esophagus, stomach, small intestine, large intestine (colon), rectum, and anus. In this portion, we'll explore some common indicators and origins of such digestive complications.

Symptoms

Even though the indicators might diverge based on the specific ailment, usual indicators linked with digestive complications may involve:

Abdominal Unease: Discomfort in the stomach or abdominal area is a frequent sign. This unease can exhibit itself in different ways - intense, cramping, or a broad sense of discomfort.

Modifications in Bowel Activities: This can involve constipation (difficult or sporadic bowel activities), diarrhea (loose, watery excrements), or a fluctuation between the two. Alterations in the hue or consistency of excrements can also imply a digestive complication.

Inflation and Gas: An excessive quantity of gas within the digestive system can instigate feelings of bloating and abdominal unease.

Nausea and Vomiting: Sensations of nausea and instances of vomiting can be indicative of a wide variety of digestive complications.

Heartburn: This manifests as a burning feeling in the chest, usually following meals, induced by stomach acid refluxing into the esophagus.

Loss of Appetite or Unanticipated Weight Loss: Modifications in appetite or unexpected reduction in weight can sometimes signify a more serious digestive complication.

Causes

Various factors can instigate the emergence of digestive complications, including:

Diet and Lifestyle: Consumption of high-fat or spicy foods, lack of physical activity, stress, and inadequate hydration can lead to many usual digestive complications, such as gastroesophageal reflux disease (GERD), peptic ulcers, and irritable bowel syndrome (IBS).

Infections: Bacterial or viral infections can lead to complications like food poisoning and gastroenteritis.

Chronic Conditions: Certain digestive complications are chronic conditions that may have an autoimmune component, such as Crohn's disease and celiac disease.

Structural Abnormalities: Complications with the structure of the GI tract can result in conditions like diverticulitis and hernias.

Genetics: Certain digestive complications, like inflammatory bowel disease and lactose intolerance, may have a genetic component.

The subsequent portion will delve into how natural remedies can be utilized to manage some of these ailments in combination with traditional medical treatments.

Herbal Remedies for Common Digestive Issues: Indigestion, Bloating, and More

The practice of employing herbal therapies to fortify digestive health has long-standing traditions. While these do not act as replacements for medical consultation or treatment, they have the potential to enhance standard treatment regimens and contribute to managing the symptoms of common digestive disturbances like indigestion, swelling, and more.

Notice: *The herbal therapies we will examine in this and the ensuing chapters may exhibit some commonalities. It's important to recognize that the same herb, depending on its intrinsic properties, could be utilized to address a wide range of conditions. Consider turmeric (curcuma longa), usually harnessed for its role in fostering digestive wellness, from calming troubled stomachs to reducing inflammation in the case of inflammatory bowel disease. Interestingly, it's also the subject of research for its prospective role in cardiac health, specifically in reducing inflammation and oxidative processes associated with atherosclerosis. Moreover, preliminary research suggests that curcumin might contribute to brain health as it can* *penetrate the blood-brain barrier and has demonstrated potential in combatting age-associated degenerative changes and mood disturbances like depression.*

Each remedy will be considered in the context of the disease in question.

Indigestion and Heartburn

Indigestion, identified by a discomfort in your stomach following a meal, and heartburn, a sensation of burning in your chest, can often be regulated with herbs like:

Peppermint (Mentha piperita): Peppermint, a highly adaptable member of the mint family, is acclaimed for its soothing influence on the gastrointestinal tract. Its primary compound, menthol, is effective in easing spasms in the GI tract, bile duct, and gallbladder. In the form of tea, it can provide relief from symptoms of indigestion, encompassing bloating, gas, and abdominal discomfort. However, people with gastroesophageal reflux disease (GERD) or hiatal hernia should abstain from peppermint as it could intensify their symptoms by causing relaxation of the lower esophageal sphincter, thus facilitating reflux of stomach acid into the esophagus.

Chamomile (Matricaria recutita): Distinguished for its tranquilizing properties, chamomile tea can be beneficial in managing indigestion. It can pacify the digestive tract, lessen inflammation, and facilitate the expulsion of gas. Additionally, its mild sedative effects can be notably advantageous when indigestion is stress or anxiety-induced, as it can help decrease stress levels, indirectly aiding in the alleviation of indigestion symptoms.

Licorice (Glycyrrhiza glabra): Licorice root is a staple in traditional medicine for addressing a variety of digestive disturbances, encompassing heartburn and stomach ulcers. Deglycyrrhizinated licorice (DGL) is a form of licorice that has been stripped of glycyrrhizin – a natural component of licorice root that can induce side effects like high blood pressure. DGL can assist in safeguarding the lining of the stomach and esophagus, mitigating symptoms of heartburn and indigestion. However, it's key to remember that prolonged usage of licorice might have side effects, hence it's prudent to consult with a healthcare professional before starting a new therapeutic regimen.

Bloating and Gas

Bloating and gas can be quite bothersome and potentially embarrassing. There are specific herbs that may provide relief:

Fennel (Foeniculum vulgare): Fennel seeds have a historical reputation in both culinary and medicinal contexts for their capacity to alleviate digestive discomfort and prevent the buildup of gas, a property known as carminative. Munching on fennel seeds or enjoying fennel tea may help dispel gas, mitigate bloating, and even ameliorate symptoms of irritable bowel syndrome (IBS). Additionally, fennel seeds contain a compound called anethole, which has antispasmodic properties and can contribute to relaxing the muscles in the gastrointestinal tract, further alleviating discomfort.

Caraway (Carum carvi): Caraway seeds, possessing a warm, sweet, and subtly peppery taste, have a history of use in traditional medicine to boost digestion. Their carminative attributes can help decrease gas and alleviate feelings of bloating or fullness. Caraway seeds can be chewed, brewed into a tea, or used as a spice in cooking to enjoy their benefits.

Ginger (Zingiber officinale): Ginger is recognized as a remedy for a variety of digestive disturbances. The root is enriched with compounds known as gingerols and shogaols, which can stimulate the expulsion of intestinal gas, thereby reducing bloating and the associated discomfort. Furthermore, ginger aids in overall digestion by promoting the movement of food and waste through the digestive system efficiently. It can be consumed as a tea, used in cooking, or even eaten raw, based on personal preference.

Constipation

Consistent bowel movements are vital for sustaining digestive health. The ensuing herbs can assist in stimulating digestion and alleviating constipation:

Senna (Senna alexandrina): The plant's leaves and pods have compounds known as sennosides, which provoke the bowel's lining and induce a laxative effect. Owing to its potency, senna should be used with caution and is usually recommended for temporary use only. Staying hydrated while using senna is vital, as it can lead to fluid loss.

Psyllium (Plantago ovata): Psyllium is a type of fiber derived from the husks of seeds from the Plantago ovata plant. Its mechanism involves absorbing water in your gut, simplifying bowel movements and making them more regular. Psyllium, with its high fiber content, can help mitigate both constipation and mild diarrhea. When using psyllium, it's crucial to drink plenty of water since it requires water absorption to function effectively.

Slippery Elm (Ulmus rubra): Known for its calming properties, it's often employed to alleviate inflammatory conditions of the digestive tract, such as gastritis and acid reflux. Regarding constipation, slippery elm acts as a demulcent, forming a slick gel that covers and soothes the intestines, facilitating easier stool passage.

Diarrhea

Herbs that can aid in managing diarrhea encompass:

Blackberry Leaf (Rubus fruticosus): Blackberry leaf is abundant in tannins, a type of astringent substances that can help tighten the tissues in the intestines. This property can help decrease excessive water loss in the stool, potentially making blackberry leaf an effective diarrhea remedy. It is usually consumed as a tea and is also available in a dried form for making decoctions or infusions.

Agrimony (Agrimonia eupatoria): Agrimony is an herb with a long-standing usage history in traditional medicine. It has astringent qualities, implying it can help tighten the gastrointestinal tract's mucous membranes. This property can assist in reducing excessive fluid loss in the stool, potentially making it an effective remedy for diarrhea. Moreover, agrimony is also known to have anti-inflammatory and antimicrobial properties. It is usually consumed as a tea or tincture. Like any herbal remedy, it's essential to consult with a healthcare professional before using it, particularly for individuals with pre-existing conditions or those on medication.

Herbals for Serious Digestive Conditions: IBS, Ulcers, etc.

While herbal therapies can provide support in managing symptoms of more severe digestive issues, they should be incorporated into a holistic treatment plan monitored by a medical professional. Here are some herbs often used for ailments such as irritable bowel syndrome (IBS), ulcers, among others:

Irritable Bowel Syndrome (IBS)

IBS is a widespread disorder impacting the large intestine and can induce an array of symptoms like cramping, abdominal pain, bloating, and alterations in bowel routines.

Peppermint (Mentha piperita): Peppermint has various active components, the most crucial for digestive health being menthol. Menthol can exert an antispasmodic effect on the muscles of the gastrointestinal (GI) tract, potentially reducing pain, bloating, and bowel irregularities associated with IBS. The typical mode of peppermint consumption for this aim is via enteric-coated peppermint oil capsules, engineered to resist digestion until they reach the intestines.

Fennel (Foeniculum vulgare): Fennel seeds possess a mix of active compounds, like anethole, fenchone, and estragole, which have antispasmodic and anti-inflammatory effects. These compounds can help mitigate IBS symptoms, particularly gas and bloating. Fennel can be consumed in the form of tea, tincture, or capsules.

Slippery Elm (Ulmus rubra): The inner bark of the slippery elm tree, known for its calming properties, is employed in herbal medicine. It contains a soluble fiber type known as mucilage. When combined with water, mucilage forms a slick gel capable of coating and soothing the intestines' lining, thus reducing inflammation and pain associated with IBS. It's typically consumed as tea, capsules, or in a powdered form mixed with water.

Peptic Ulcers

Peptic ulcers are lesions that form in the stomach, upper small intestine, or esophagus lining.

Licorice (Glycyrrhiza glabra): Deglycyrrhizinated licorice (DGL), which is licorice from which a potentially harmful substance has been removed, is often used for this purpose. It is believed that DGL aids in increasing the number of mucus-secreting cells in the digestive tract, forming a protective layer over the stomach lining and facilitating ulcer healing. DGL is typically consumed in the form of chewable tablets.

Marshmallow Root (Althaea officinalis): Marshmallow root is another time-honored remedy for digestive issues, including ulcers. Similar to DGL, it is presumed to work by boosting mucus production, thereby protecting the stomach and intestines lining. Marshmallow root can be consumed as a tea, in capsules, or as a tincture.

Cabbage (Brassica oleracea): Although not a herb in the traditional sense, cabbage has been employed for centuries as a natural remedy for peptic ulcers. The juice of the cabbage is especially rich in glutamine, an amino acid that encourages the growth and regeneration of the stomach lining cells, potentially aiding in ulcer healing. Consuming fresh cabbage juice is the typical method to benefit from this effect.

Inflammatory Bowel Disease (IBD)

IBD, encompassing conditions like Crohn's disease and ulcerative colitis, involves enduring inflammation within the digestive system.

Boswellia (Boswellia serrata): Also known as Indian frankincense, Boswellia has long been utilized in Ayurvedic medicine. Renowned for its anti-inflammatory effects, due to active compounds named boswellic acids, initial research points towards Boswellia potentially helping mitigate inflammation in individuals with IBD. The resin extracted from the Boswellia tree is usually ingested in the form of capsules or tablets.

Slippery Elm (Ulmus rubra): As stated earlier, Slippery Elm is employed for its calming effects. It forms a slick gel when mixed with water, serving as a protective shield along the digestive tract lining, possibly easing symptoms tied to IBD, like inflammation and abdominal pain. Slippery Elm is usually consumed orally as a powder, which can be mixed with water or made into a gruel.

Further Herbs for Gastrointestinal Disease Prevention

Dandelion (Taraxacum officinale): The roots and leaves of this plant are abundant in inulin, a kind of fiber that acts as nourishment for beneficial gut bacteria, encouraging their proliferation and activity. This renders dandelion an excellent prebiotic, potentially improving digestion, reducing bloating and constipation, and enhancing nutrient absorption. Dandelion can be consumed in the form of tea, tincture, or capsules.

Marshmallow Root (Althaea officinalis): Marshmallow root is rich in mucilage, a gel-like substance that coats and shields the digestive tract lining. This makes it highly beneficial for conditions causing inflammation and irritation in the gut, such as gastritis and acid reflux. The calming effects of marshmallow root can help alleviate pain, inflammation, and other symptoms linked to these conditions. Marshmallow root is typically consumed as a tea or in capsule form.

Aloe Vera (Aloe barbadensis): Recognized for its soothing and healing properties, the gel extracted from the aloe vera plant can help decrease inflammation and encourage healing within the digestive tract. This makes it particularly beneficial for conditions like gastritis and ulcers. Aloe vera can be consumed as a juice or in gel form, but it's crucial to ensure that the product is designed for internal use.

Incorporating these herbs into your daily routine can help boost gut health and digestion. However, it's always recommended to consult a medical professional before starting any new herbal treatment, as they can interact with medications and present their own side effects. Moreover, gut health is intricate and influenced by various factors, so it's crucial to maintain a balanced diet, regular exercise, and stress management for optimal digestive health.

Chapter Six: Respiratory Conditions

Respiratory issues impact the air passages and various lung components. This section offers a summary of the symptoms and causes of prevalent respiratory conditions to form a foundation for comprehending how herbal treatments can aid respiratory wellbeing.

Asthma

Asthma is a persistent issue affecting the lung's airways, leading to inflammation and constriction. Symptoms encompass wheezing, breathlessness, chest constriction, and coughing.

Roots: Various factors can trigger asthma, such as allergens (like dust mites, animal fur, and pollen), respiratory infections, physical exertion, frigid air, and stress.

Chronic Obstructive Pulmonary Disease (COPD)

COPD is a lasting inflammatory lung disease that obstructs the airflow from the lungs. The primary symptoms are breathlessness, overproduction of sputum, and a lasting cough.

Roots: Prolonged exposure to irritating gases or particulate matter, mainly from cigarette smoke, is the primary cause of COPD. Long-term exposure to air pollution and inhalation of dust and chemicals in certain professions can also contribute to COPD development.

Bronchitis

Bronchitis is an inflammation of your bronchial tubes' lining, which facilitates air transport to and from your lungs. Symptoms include a cough with mucus, breathlessness, chest constriction, and tiredness.

Roots: Viruses, typically the same ones causing a common cold or the flu, are the main cause of bronchitis. Smoking and exposure to specific pollutants can also lead to bronchitis.

Pneumonia

Pneumonia is an infection in one or both lungs that inflames the air sacs and might fill them with fluid or pus. Symptoms encompass a cough with phlegm or pus, fever, chills, and difficulty breathing.

Roots: Pneumonia can be triggered by a variety of organisms, including bacteria, viruses, and fungi. It often occurs after a cold or the flu when your immune system might be weakened.

Herbal Remedies for Common Respiratory Ailments: Cold, Cough, and Asthma

The respiratory system can often be susceptible to infections and disorders that can interrupt our everyday routines. Although contemporary medicine provides numerous solutions for these problems, an extensive array of herbal alternatives can also provide relief and aid recovery. In this section, we will explore some of these botanical choices for prevalent respiratory issues like colds, coughs, and asthma.

Common Cold

The common cold is a viral affliction primarily impacting the nose and throat. Symptoms involve a runny nose, sneezing, and blockage. The following plants can help manage these signs:

Echinacea (Echinacea purpurea): Indigenous Americans have traditionally used Echinacea to alleviate various health problems, and it remains a sought-after plant in the realm of complementary and alternative therapies today. Echinacea is thought to strengthen the immune system and diminish symptoms of sicknesses like the common cold and the flu. Some elements of echinacea, like polysaccharides, alkylamides, and chicoric acid, have demonstrated immunomodulatory effects, enhancing the body's defenses against infections. Echinacea can be enjoyed as a tea, tincture, or capsule.

Elderberry (Sambucus nigra): Elderberries are small, dark fruits that offer substantial health benefits. These berries are abundant in antioxidants and vitamins, including vitamin C, that strengthen the immune system and foster overall wellness. Elderberries also contain anthocyanins, boasting anti-inflammatory and antiviral attributes. This makes them particularly potent at combatting cold and flu symptoms. Elderberry is often consumed as a syrup but can also be enjoyed as a tea or in capsule form.

Garlic: Garlic is home to a compound known as allicin, possessing potent medicinal attributes, including antioxidant, antimicrobial, and immune-strengthening effects. Regular garlic consumption can enhance the immune system's functionality, lowering the likelihood of falling ill. Garlic is most powerful when eaten fresh, but it can also be consumed in capsule form or used in cooking.

Cough

A cough can be a response to a tickling sensation in the throat, the body's reaction to foreign particles, or an indicator of a more significant problem. Here are some plants that can help relieve coughs:

Marshmallow root (Althaea officinalis): Marshmallow root is a plant originating from Europe, Western Asia, and Northern Africa. It's been used in traditional healing for millennia to treat a range of conditions, including coughs and sore throats. The root of the marshmallow plant contains a type of soluble fiber called mucilage. When mixed with water, mucilage forms a slick gel that can coat and soothe the throat and stomach lining, reducing irritation and inflammation. Marshmallow root can be consumed as a tea, tincture, or in capsule form.

Licorice Root (Glycyrrhiza glabra): Licorice root, fondly known as sweet root, is a flavourful plant that has found its way into our kitchens and health remedies for hundreds of years. Besides its celebrated role in soothing digestive troubles, licorice is an efficient expectorant, assisting the body in loosening and clearing away excess mucus. It also offers anti-inflammatory effects that can aid in easing a sore or irritated throat. Licorice can be enjoyed as a tea or incorporated into a lozenge that soothes the throat.

Thyme (Thymus vulgaris): Thyme, a fragrant herb with minute leaves, is not just a staple in our spice racks but also a formidable healing agent. It is enriched with two health-promoting compounds, thymol and carvacrol, both renowned for their antimicrobial and antispasmodic properties. These qualities make thyme a powerful ally for calming coughs and addressing other respiratory concerns. Thyme's antispasmodic activity aids in relaxing the airways, enhancing the productivity of coughs and potentially mitigating the symptoms of conditions like bronchitis. Thyme is typically consumed as a tea or syrup to alleviate coughs and soothe sore throats.

Asthma: Asthma is a condition where your airways constrict and become inflamed, potentially producing extra mucus. This can lead to breathing difficulties, coughing, a whistling sound upon exhaling (wheezing), and shortness of breath.

Ginkgo Biloba (Ginkgo biloba): Ginkgo is abundant in powerful antioxidants, specifically flavonoids and terpenoids, which help to fight against oxidative stress and inflammation, two crucial factors in the manifestation of asthma. Generally consumed as a tea or supplement, Ginkgo may help in improving breathing and decreasing the frequency and intensity of asthma attacks. Nevertheless, studies are still ongoing, and more evidence is required to completely understand Ginkgo's role in treating asthma.

Turmeric (Curcuma longa): Curcumin, the active component in turmeric, has been identified to obstruct the release of inflammatory cells within the body, which can assist in managing the inflammation related to asthma. Turmeric can be incorporated into our diets in several ways, but for respiratory concerns, it's often taken as a supplement or brewed in teas.

Lobelia (Lobelia inflata): Lobelia is perceived to work as a bronchodilator, potentially relaxing the bronchial muscles and opening up the airways, enabling easier breathing. It's also considered to work as an expectorant, aiding in clearing mucus from the lungs. Despite its potential advantages, Lobelia can be toxic in excessive quantities, so it should be used under the guidance of a healthcare professional.

Herbs for Chronic Respiratory Diseases: COPD and Allergies

Long-term respiratory illnesses, such as Chronic Obstructive Pulmonary Disease (COPD) and allergies, can considerably affect an individual's lifestyle. While these health conditions necessitate expert diagnosis and medical intervention, specific herbs can complement standard treatment by relieving symptoms and boosting overall well-being. Let's examine how herbal solutions can contribute to managing these long-term respiratory ailments.

Chronic Obstructive Pulmonary Disease (COPD)

COPD is a designation given to a collection of progressive lung diseases, which include emphysema, chronic bronchitis, and non-reversible asthma. Symptoms often manifest as breathlessness, frequent bouts of coughing, a sensation of chest tightness, and wheezing. Here are a few herbs that might augment COPD treatment:

Astragalus (Astragalus membranaceus): Astragalus is a flowering perennial plant that originates from the northern and eastern regions of China, as well as Mongolia and Korea. It has been a cornerstone of traditional Chinese medicine for centuries due to its immune-enhancing and anti-inflammatory properties. In relation to Chronic Obstructive Pulmonary Disease (COPD), astragalus is believed to aid in mitigating lung inflammation, bolstering lung function, and strengthening the immune system. Some studies suggest that astragalus may offer protective effects on lung injury by modulating immune responses, although further research is required in this domain. Astragalus can be enjoyed as a tea, encapsulated, or in tincture form.

Eucalyptus (Eucalyptus globulus): Eucalyptus, a tree species native to Australia, has had its essential oil used for centuries in traditional medicine as a remedy for respiratory ailments. The primary component of eucalyptus oil, cineole, possesses anti-inflammatory, pain-relieving, and mucolytic properties, implying it can aid in mucus breakdown and airway clearance. For those living with COPD, inhaling eucalyptus oil might assist in alleviating congestion, enhancing breathing, and reducing the inflammation that exacerbates COPD symptoms. However, eucalyptus oil should be administered with care, as it can induce breathing difficulties in certain individuals, particularly when applied directly to the nasal area or used in excess quantities.

Ginger (Zingiber officinale): A research paper published in the American Journal of Respiratory Cell and Molecular Biology suggested that compounds found in ginger helped to relax the airway smooth muscle, which could potentially enhance breathing for individuals with COPD. Ginger can be consumed in a myriad of forms, such as fresh, dried, as a tea, or encapsulated.

Allergies

Allergies arise when the body's immune system exhibits an exaggerated response to environmental substances like pollen, dust mites, or specific foods. Common symptoms include sneezing, itchiness, skin rash, and breathing difficulties. The following herbs can aid in controlling allergy symptoms:

Nettle (Urtica dioica): Commonly known as stinging nettle, this perennial blooming plant has been employed in medicinal applications for numerous centuries. It boasts a diverse range of nutrients, including vitamins A, C, K, and various B vitamins, along with minerals such as calcium, iron, magnesium, phosphorus, potassium, and sodium. Nettle is recognized as a natural antihistamine due to its capacity to inhibit the body's production of histamines, chemicals your body generates during an allergic response. By preventing histamine production, nettle can assist in alleviating allergy symptoms like sneezing, a runny nose, and itchy, water-filled eyes. Nettle can be taken in several forms, such as teas, tinctures, and capsules.

Butterbur (Petasites hybridus): Butterbur is a plant that thrives in wet, marshy terrain, with its leaves traditionally serving as a natural remedy for various ailments including migraines, stomach spasms, coughs, allergies, and asthma. In terms of allergies, multiple studies indicate that butterbur extract can match the effectiveness of some over-the-counter antihistamines for relieving nasal symptoms. It's believed to function by mitigating inflammation and impeding leukotrienes, chemicals that ignite allergic reactions. Butterbur can be consumed as teas, tinctures, or capsules.

Quercetin: Quercetin is a type of flavonoid, a plant pigment that gives many fruits and vegetables their colors. It possesses antioxidant and anti-inflammatory properties, and is thought to aid in reducing the release of histamines. This can help to diminish allergic reactions including hives, watery eyes, a runny nose, and swelling. Quercetin is found in a variety of foods including onions, apples, berries, and green tea, but can also be taken in supplement form.

COPD and severe allergies are significant health conditions that can lead to critical complications if not properly managed. Herbal solutions should be regarded as a supportive measure to conventional medical treatment and should always be administered under the guidance of a healthcare provider. Moreover, lifestyle modifications such as ceasing smoking, maintaining a healthy weight, and regular physical exercise can considerably enhance the quality of life for those living with chronic respiratory disorders.

Chapter Seven: Cardiovascular Health

Cardiovascular wellness encapsulates the overall health of the heart and the network of blood vessels. A variety of conditions can influence cardiovascular wellbeing, leading to substantial effects on one's overall health. Understanding these conditions forms the basis for appreciating how herbal remedies can contribute to cardiovascular wellness.

Hypertension (Elevated Blood Pressure)

Hypertension is a state in which the pressure of blood against the arterial walls is persistently elevated. Over the long run, this can culminate in severe health complications, such as cardiac disease and stroke.

Causative Factors: Elements like aging, family medical history, high-sodium diet, insufficient physical activity, obesity, stress, and certain underlying health conditions can contribute to hypertension.

Coronary Artery Disease (CAD)

CAD is the most prevalent type of cardiac disease. It transpires when the coronary arteries responsible for delivering blood to the heart muscle harden and narrow due to plaque build-up on the interior walls or lining of these arteries (atherosclerosis).

Causative Factors: Factors that contribute to atherosclerosis encompass high cholesterol levels in the blood, tobacco usage, insulin resistance or diabetes, and high blood pressure.

Heart Failure

Heart failure, otherwise known as congestive heart failure, develops when the heart muscle doesn't circulate blood as efficiently as it should. Conditions like narrowed arteries or high blood pressure slowly leave the heart too weakened or rigid to effectively fill and pump.

Causative Factors: Numerous conditions can lead to heart failure, including coronary artery disease, elevated blood pressure, defective heart valves, heart muscle damage, among others.

Arrhythmia

Arrhythmia signifies abnormal heart rhythms. The heart may beat too slowly, too rapidly, or irregularly. Arrhythmias can span from benign to life-threatening.

Causative Factors: Arrhythmias can be attributed to many factors, including heart disease, high blood pressure, alterations in the heart muscle, injury resulting from a heart attack, and other health conditions.

Peripheral Artery Disease (PAD)

PAD is a circulatory condition where constricted blood vessels decrease blood flow to the limbs. PAD typically affects the arteries in the legs, but it can also impact the arteries that transport blood from the heart to the head, arms, kidneys, and stomach.

Causitive Factors: Atherosclerosis is the most prevalent cause of PAD, but it can also be provoked by blood clots or inflammation in the blood vessels.

Herbal Remedies for Common Cardiovascular Issues

While traditional medicine provides potent solutions for these conditions, a variety of herbal remedies can contribute to overall cardiovascular wellbeing and potentially aid in managing these health issues.

Hypertension (Elevated Blood Pressure)

Hypertension is a state where the pressure of the blood against the arterial walls is too high. If not effectively managed, it can culminate in severe complications such as cardiac disease and stroke. Here are some botanicals that can assist in managing hypertension:

Hawthorn (Crataegus spp.): Hawthorn is a variety of plant utilized for medicinal purposes for hundreds of years, especially in Europe and Asia. It's often employed for heart-associated conditions and is thought to enhance cardiovascular wellbeing by expanding blood vessels, enhancing blood flow, and assisting the heart in pumping more efficiently. Its berries, leaves, and blossoms are rich in antioxidants, including flavonoids and oligomeric proanthocyanidins, which can aid in safeguarding the heart from damage. Some research suggests that hawthorn may help lower blood pressure in individuals with hypertension, although additional research is necessary. Hawthorn can be taken as a tea, in capsule form, or as a tincture.

Garlic (Allium sativum): Notable for its potent aroma and flavor, which stems from its sulfur compounds. One of these compounds, allicin, is thought to possess significant medicinal properties, including the ability to lower blood pressure. Several studies propose that consuming garlic can assist in lowering blood pressure, especially in individuals with hypertension. Garlic can be consumed in its raw form or as a supplement in tablet or capsule form.

Celery seeds (Apium graveolens): Celery seeds are derived from the flowers of the celery plant, a common vegetable worldwide. In traditional Chinese medicine, celery seeds have been long employed to treat a variety of cardiovascular issues, including hypertension. Contemporary research suggests that specific compounds in celery seeds may have blood pressure-lowering effects. These compounds are thought to work by relaxing the muscles in and around the walls of arteries and veins, aiding in blood vessel dilation and reducing blood pressure. Celery seeds can be consumed as a spice, in teas, or as a supplement in capsule form.

Bear in mind, lifestyle alterations such as a nutritious diet, consistent exercise, moderating alcohol and sodium intake, maintaining a healthy weight, and managing stress are also crucial in managing high blood pressure.

Atherosclerosis

Atherosclerosis encompasses the accumulation of fats, cholesterol, and additional substances in and along the arterial walls (plaques), potentially impeding blood flow.

Here are a few botanicals that might aid in the management of atherosclerosis:

Ginkgo Biloba (Ginkgo biloba): The leaves of the Ginkgo tree are loaded with potent antioxidants that counter the oxidative stress associated with numerous chronic diseases, encompassing heart disease and atherosclerosis. These antioxidants, inclusive of flavonoids and terpenoids, are considered to aid in safeguarding the heart and blood vessels from oxidative damage. Some research implies that Ginkgo Biloba might also aid in enhancing blood flow and inhibiting blood clots, further contributing to its potential advantages for cardiac health. Ginkgo Biloba can be consumed as tea, in capsule form, or as a tincture.

Turmeric (Curcuma longa): By reducing inflammation and oxidation, curcumin may assist in protection against the development and progression of atherosclerosis. Curcumin has also been demonstrated to improve the function of the endothelium, the lining of the blood vessels, crucial for cardiac health. Turmeric can be consumed in its spice form, as a tea, or in capsule form as a supplement.

Ginger (Zingiber officinale): The potent anti-inflammatory compounds in ginger, known as gingerols, might aid in reducing inflammation in the blood vessels, a crucial factor in atherosclerosis. Furthermore, some research suggests that ginger might also aid in lowering cholesterol and preventing blood clotting, two additional factors that can contribute to atherosclerosis. Ginger can be consumed fresh, dried, as a spice, in tea, or in capsule form as a supplement.

Other Botanicals for Cardiac Health

Certain herbs have a more generalized impact on cardiovascular health and could potentially assist with diverse cardiovascular conditions:

Flaxseeds (Linum usitatissimum): Flaxseeds, also referred to as linseeds, are minute seeds that stem from the Linum usitatissimum plant. They're recognized for their brown or golden hue and their distinctive, nutty flavor. A widely recognized nutritional powerhouse, flaxseeds have multiple health advantages primarily due to their high content of dietary fiber and alpha-linolenic acid (ALA), a type of omega-3 fatty acid.

The dietary fiber present in flaxseeds not only aids in digestion, reducing constipation, but it also assists in weight management by promoting feelings of satiety. Moreover, it assists in controlling blood sugar levels, thus potentially beneficial for individuals with diabetes.

In terms of cardiovascular health, flaxseeds are particularly beneficial. They are a rich source of omega-3 fatty acids, which have been extensively researched for their heart-healthy properties. ALA, the specific omega-3 present in flaxseeds, can decrease inflammation, lower elevated blood pressure, and reduce the buildup of plaques in the arteries. By doing so, flaxseeds can aid in lowering LDL, or "bad," cholesterol levels and decrease the risk of heart disease.

Green Tea (Camellia sinensis): Green tea, originating from the Camellia sinensis plant, is among the most popular drinks worldwide, particularly celebrated for its health-enhancing qualities. This is mainly due to its abundant content of bioactive components like polyphenols and catechins, which have strong antioxidant characteristics.

Polyphenols are natural compounds found in numerous plants, inclusive of tea leaves. They are potent antioxidants that safeguard the body's cells against damage from free radicals, which can lead to chronic ailments such as cancer and heart disease. Catechins, a type of polyphenol especially abundant in green tea, exhibit not only antioxidant capabilities but also anti-inflammatory and anticarcinogenic properties.

Frequent consumption of green tea has been linked to several health advantages, particularly concerning cardiovascular health. The catechins in green tea can aid in lowering blood pressure and reducing LDL cholesterol levels. They operate by inhibiting the absorption of cholesterol and enhancing its excretion from the body, aiding in preventing the accumulation of plaques in the arteries. This, in turn, decreases the risk of heart disease and stroke. Furthermore, the natural compounds in green tea can also aid in enhancing blood vessel function and promoting fat burning, making it advantageous for weight management.

Arjuna (Terminalia arjuna): Arjuna is a sizable deciduous tree native to India, where it has been used extensively in Ayurvedic medicine for centuries, especially for cardiovascular conditions. The bark of the Arjuna tree, which is abundant in saponins, natural steroids, flavonoids, and other bioactive compounds, is most commonly used for medicinal purposes.

The therapeutic benefits of Arjuna on the heart are numerous. It is thought to enhance the function of the cardiac muscle, which contributes to the heart's ability to pump blood more efficiently. This can lead to improved heart function, particularly in those with heart disease or heart failure.

Arjuna also contains an abundance of antioxidants, which can combat oxidative stress and free radical damage in the body. This is critical for heart health because oxidative stress can lead to inflammation and the development of atherosclerotic plaques, both of which can contribute to heart disease. The anti-inflammatory properties of Arjuna further enhance its cardiovascular benefits, as chronic inflammation is often associated with heart disease.

Moreover, Arjuna is renowned for its blood-thinning properties, which can aid in preventing blood clots and reducing the risk of heart attacks and strokes. Additionally, it may help to lower high blood pressure and cholesterol levels, further contributing to its role in maintaining heart health. Despite these potential benefits, more robust clinical trials are needed to confirm the effectiveness of Arjuna for these uses.

Chapter Eight: Mental and Emotional Health

Mental and emotional wellness is a fundamental component of our total health. It's intrinsically linked with our physical wellness, and overlooking one can have profound implications on the other. Let's delve into some of the most prevalent mental and emotional health disorders.

Depression is an emotional health disorder identified by consistent feelings of sorrow, despair, and a lack of enthusiasm in everyday tasks. It is a widespread but grave disorder that impacts how an individual feels, thinks, and conducts themselves, often resulting in a multitude of physical and emotional complications.

Anxiety disorders represent a set of psychological health disorders defined by sensations of worry and fear. These feelings might prompt physical symptoms, such as an accelerated heartbeat and trembling. Varieties of anxiety disorders encompass generalized anxiety disorder, panic disorder, and diverse phobia-related disorders.

Post-Traumatic Stress Disorder (PTSD) is a psychological health condition initiated by a horrifying event, either through experiencing or observing it. Symptoms might encompass vivid recollections, nightmares, severe anxiety, and uncontrollable thoughts concerning the event.

Stress-Related Disorders can result in numerous mental and physical health problems when it becomes chronic. These can range from sleep disorders to cardiovascular diseases. Managing stress is, therefore, crucial for comprehensive health.

Attention-Deficit/Hyperactivity Disorder (ADHD) is a disorder characterized by enduring patterns of distraction, hyperactivity, and impulsiveness that interfere with functioning or development.

Bipolar Disorder, previously known as manic depression, is a mental health condition that leads to severe mood swings that incorporate emotional highs (mania or hypomania) and lows (depression).

Herbal Remedies for Stress, Anxiety, and Depression

Numerous botanicals have been traditionally utilized to support mental wellness:

St. John's Wort (Hypericum perforatum): This is a perennial plant that thrives in wilderness areas across the globe. St. John's Wort is acclaimed for its potential mental wellness benefits. It has been utilized for hundreds of years to manage mood disorders, especially depression. Clinical research endorses its use for mild to moderate depression. Its mechanism of action seems to inhibit the reabsorption of the neurotransmitters serotonin, dopamine, and norepinephrine, thereby amplifying their presence in the brain.

Notwithstanding its potential advantages, St. John's Wort should be used prudently due to its interactions with numerous medications. This is because it can influence the liver enzymes responsible for metabolizing medications, potentially modifying their effectiveness.

Ashwagandha (Withania somnifera): Also known as Indian ginseng or winter cherry, Ashwagandha is a core herb in Ayurveda, an ancient form of Indian medicine. It is recognized as an adaptogen, suggesting it can aid your body in managing stress. It provides a multitude of health benefits owing to its abundant content of withanolides, a group of steroidal lactones, which contribute to its medicinal properties.

Ashwagandha is reputed to empower the body to conserve and maintain vital energy throughout the day while fostering deep, restorative sleep at night. It can potentially lower cortisol levels, a hormone elevated during chronic stress. Moreover, it has been studied for its potential to lessen anxiety and depression, boost brain function, and even combat inflammation and oxidative stress.

Passionflower (Passiflora incarnata): Native to southeastern parts of the Americas, passionflower is recognized for its enchanting flowers and medicinal properties. Traditionally, it has been used as a tranquilizing herb to manage conditions related to anxiety and insomnia.

The soothing and sedative effects of passionflower are believed to stem from its content of flavonoids, known to interact with the gamma-aminobutyric acid (GABA) system in the brain, a system that helps regulate mood. By augmenting the levels of GABA in the brain, passionflower can diminish the activity of certain brain cells, inciting relaxation and fostering better sleep.

Lemon Balm (Melissa officinalis): Belonging to the mint family, lemon balm is a herb indigenous to parts of Europe and the Mediterranean. It's widely appreciated for its calming effects and its potential to boost cognitive function.

The herb contains various compounds, including rosmarinic acid and triterpenoids, which have demonstrated anti-stress, anti-anxiety, and neuroprotective properties. Regular consumption of lemon balm has been associated with reduced stress and anxiety, mood enhancement, and improved cognitive performance.

Rhodiola (Rhodiola Rosea): Rhodiola is recognized as an adaptogen, assisting the body in acclimating to various forms of stress, be they physical, chemical, or environmental. It boasts over 140 active ingredients, with rosavin and salidroside being the two most potent. These active constituents are considered instrumental in the plant's capacity to mitigate stress symptoms such as weariness, burnout, and worry.

Numerous scientific investigations corroborate these uses. For instance, Rhodiola has been observed to refine the body's stress response by modulating crucial brain chemicals like serotonin and norepinephrine, as well as the naturally occurring euphoria-inducing opioids known as beta-endorphins. This can culminate in improved cognitive performance, particularly during times of heightened stress.

Lavender (Lavandula angustifolia): Easily recognizable by its charming floral fragrance, lavender is a blooming plant in the mint family. It's native to the Old World, found from Cape Verde and the Canary Islands to Europe, northern and eastern Africa, the Mediterranean, southwest Asia, and southeast India.

Renowned for its soothing and tranquilizing properties, lavender has been used over centuries to alleviate anxiety, sleep disorders, and depression. Its active constituents, including linalool and linalyl acetate, have potent mood-balancing and sedative properties.

In the realm of aromatherapy, the inhalation of lavender essential oil is frequently employed to foster relaxation and sleep. Furthermore, oral lavender supplements have demonstrated promising results in managing anxiety and associated sleep disturbances. However, it's crucial to underscore that oral consumption should always be under the oversight of a medical professional, as lavender oil can be toxic if ingested in excessive quantities.

Herbs for Improving Memory and Cognitive Function

Our intellectual abilities include aspects like memory, focus, perception, reasoning, problem-solving, and decision-making. These capabilities play a crucial role in our everyday lives, and their deterioration can have a notable impact on our lifestyle. Various herbs have been traditionally utilized to bolster memory and cognitive function. While they don't serve as a cure for cognitive impairment or neurodegenerative conditions, they can aid brain health and potentially enhance intellectual performance.

Bacopa Monnieri (Brahmi): Bacopa Monnieri, often referred to as Brahmi, is a sprawling herb indigenous to the wetlands of southern and Eastern India, Australia, Europe, Africa, Asia, and North and South America. It holds a significant place in Ayurvedic medicine, admired for its potential to boost brain function.

Bacopa Monnieri is primarily recognized for its properties that enhance cognition. It has been broadly utilized to augment memory, concentration, and learning capabilities. Its influence on brain health is mainly attributed to a set of saponins called bacosides.

These bacosides are thought to mend damaged neurons and optimize nerve impulse transmission.

Research corroborates these uses. For instance, several studies indicate that supplementing with Bacopa Monnieri can accelerate information processing, curtail reaction times, and improve memory in healthy adults. The herb's antioxidants also contribute to safeguarding the brain from free radical damage.

Gotu Kola (Centella asiatica): Known as Centella asiatica, Gotu Kola is a perennial plant indigenous to the wetlands of Asia. It has been used in traditional Chinese, Indonesian, and Ayurvedic medicine for centuries to treat an array of conditions.

This herb has been credited for boosting brain function, enhancing memory and intellect, and uplifting mood. The active compounds in Gotu Kola, known as triterpenoids, appear to reduce anxiety and boost mental function in mice, suggesting potential similar benefits in humans.

It has also been employed to manage neurodegenerative conditions like Alzheimer's due to its ability to regenerate brain cells. However, while animal and lab studies hint at potential cognitive benefits and effects on Alzheimer's disease, more human research is required to validate these effects.

Ginseng (Panax ginseng): Ginseng is a traditional medicinal herb native to Eastern Asia and North America. Its health advantages stem from its root, which can be consumed in a variety of forms – fresh, dried, powdered, or as tea. The two primary types are Panax (or Korean) ginseng and American ginseng, with Panax ginseng being the most studied variant.

For centuries, it has been used to enhance brain functions such as memory, behavior, and mood. Ginsenosides, the active compounds in ginseng, exhibit neuroprotective effects, encouraging neurogenesis and shielding the brain against free radical damage.

Clinical research supports ginseng's cognitive-enhancing effects. For instance, it has been observed to enhance intellectual performance and alleviate feelings of mental fatigue. It may also hold potential benefits for managing Alzheimer's disease, with research suggesting it could improve cognitive performance in Alzheimer's patients, although more research is required to validate these findings.

Promoting Relaxation and Sleep with Herbs

Sleep is integral for our holistic wellbeing. It provides the much-needed downtime for our bodies to recuperate and plays a pivotal role in our brain's capacity to learn and retain information. Sleep disturbances are a common issue for many, and persistent sleep deficiency can lead to significant health repercussions. Certain herbs have been traditionally utilized to encourage relaxation and sleep. Let's delve into some of them:

Magnolia Bark (Magnolia officinalis): Extracted from the tree bearing the same name, Magnolia Bark has been a mainstay in traditional Chinese medicine for hundreds of years. It's been used for a plethora of health benefits, spanning from managing anxiety to treating allergies and asthma.

The bark houses several bioactive compounds, including magnolol and honokiol, which possess neuroprotective and anxiolytic properties. These compounds directly interact with the gamma-aminobutyric acid (GABA) receptors in the brain, fostering relaxation and mitigating stress. GABA is a neurotransmitter that restrains the activity of neurons, producing a calming effect.

Research suggests that Magnolia Bark may enhance sleep and relaxation by increasing the duration of non-REM sleep. Furthermore, its potential to reduce cortisol, a stress hormone, may further bolster healthy sleep patterns.

Valerian (Valeriana officinalis): Valerian is a blooming plant, native to Europe and parts of Asia, the roots of which are recognized for their medicinal properties. Its use as a medicinal herb dates back to at least the era of ancient Greece and Rome, where it was used to manage insomnia, nervousness, tremors, headaches, and stress.

Valerian root incorporates several compounds that may facilitate sleep and alleviate anxiety, including valerenic acid, isovaleric acid, and an array of antioxidants. Valerenic acid is known to obstruct the breakdown of GABA in the brain, leading to sensations of peace and tranquility.

Often ingested in capsule or tincture format, valerian root can also be brewed as a tea. Clinical research vouches for its use for insomnia and other sleep disorders, citing enhanced sleep quality and ease of falling asleep.

California Poppy (Eschscholzia californica): The California Poppy, recognized as the state flower of California, has been utilized by Native American tribes for its calming and relaxing properties. The plant houses various alkaloids, including protopine and allocryptopine, which are believed to contribute to its medicinal properties.

Its sedative characteristics make it a popular natural remedy for insomnia, anxiety, and nervous tension. Beyond promoting sleep and relaxation, California poppy is also used to moderate mood swings and mild instances of anxiety. Despite its potential benefits, more research is needed to fully comprehend the mechanisms of California poppy's effects on sleep and anxiety.

Chapter Nine: Skin and Hair Health

The health of our skin and hair play a pivotal role in our overall wellness. They act as our body's frontline soldiers, safeguarding against environmental adversities. However, numerous factors can give rise to a variety of skin and hair conditions. Let's delve into some of the prevalent conditions that can compromise skin and hair health.

Acne

Also referred to as acne vulgaris, acne is a widespread skin condition that transpires when hair follicles embedded under the skin are obstructed by sebum (a bodily-produced oily substance) and dead skin cells. This blockage results in the creation of varying types of pimples or acne lesions, encompassing whiteheads, blackheads, cysts, nodules, and pustules.

While acne predominantly impacts adolescents undergoing hormonal fluctuations during puberty, it can manifest at any stage of life. Elements contributing to acne development encompass hormonal changes, stress, certain medications, a diet high in processed sugars, and genetic factors. Acne can induce emotional distress and scar the skin, but a variety of treatments can effectively manage the condition.

Eczema (Atopic Dermatitis)

Eczema, more precisely atopic dermatitis, is a long-term, inflammatory skin disorder leading to red, dry, and itchy skin. Its incidence is highest in children, but it can afflict individuals at any age. The cause of atopic dermatitis is a fusion of genetic, immune, and environmental factors. The condition tends to periodically flare up and then ease, with some people experiencing symptoms consistently.

Atopic dermatitis is commonly linked with other allergic disorders like asthma and hay fever. Treatment primarily revolves around skin hydration, inflammation reduction, and symptom management.

Psoriasis

Psoriasis is a disease triggered by the immune system, resulting in elevated, red, scaly patches on the skin. These patches are typically found on the elbows, knees, and scalp but can emerge anywhere on the body. The cause of psoriasis is multifaceted, with genetic factors and immune system irregularities playing substantial roles.

In individuals with psoriasis, skin cells multiply much faster than normal—up to ten times quicker—leading to a buildup of cells on the skin's surface. Psoriasis is linked with other severe health conditions, such as diabetes, heart disease, and depression.

Rosacea

Rosacea is a chronic, inflammatory skin condition predominantly affecting the face. It's characterized by redness, swelling, visible blood vessels, and sometimes, small, red, pus-filled bumps. The precise cause of rosacea remains elusive, but it may be due to a blend of hereditary and environmental factors.

While there's no cure for rosacea, treatments can manage and mitigate the signs and symptoms. Triggers that may instigate a flare-up vary among individuals but can include spicy foods, alcohol, emotional stress, and hot weather.

Alopecia Areata

Alopecia areata is an autoimmune condition in which the immune system targets the hair follicles, resulting in hair loss. The hair loss may appear in patches or involve the entire scalp (termed alopecia totalis) or even the entire body (known as alopecia universalis). This condition affects both genders and can manifest at any time; however, most instances occur before reaching 30 years of age.

While the precise cause of alopecia areata remains unknown, it is thought to involve a genetic predisposition and an environmental trigger. It's commonly linked with other autoimmune conditions like thyroid disease or vitiligo. Although there's no known cure for alopecia areata, treatments exist that can expedite hair regrowth and avert future hair loss.

Dandruff and Seborrheic Dermatitis

Dandruff is a scalp condition characterized by excessive shedding of dead skin cells from the scalp. It often presents as white flakes visible in the hair and on the shoulders. While it is neither contagious nor harmful, it can be embarrassing and occasionally difficult to manage. The exact cause of dandruff remains unclear, but it might be linked to an overgrowth of yeast-like fungus, infrequent shampooing, sensitivity to hair products, or dry skin.

Seborrheic dermatitis represents a more serious form of dandruff. It is a prevalent skin disease primarily affecting areas of the skin rich in sebum glands, such as the scalp, face, chest, and back. Symptoms include redness, swelling, itching, and flaky scales. The exact cause of seborrheic dermatitis is unclear, but factors such as a yeast living on the skin, stress, cold and dry weather, and certain medical conditions can heighten the risk.

Contact Dermatitis

Contact dermatitis represents a skin inflammation type that arises from contact with allergens or irritants. Two primary types exist: irritant contact dermatitis and allergic contact dermatitis. The former is caused by substances like solvents or detergents that damage the skin's outer layer, while the latter is caused by allergens like nickel or poison ivy, triggering an allergic reaction. Symptoms may include redness, itching, swelling, and sometimes blisters and burning. The best prevention involves avoiding the cause of the reaction.

Hives (Urticaria)

Also known as urticaria, hives are red, itchy, raised welts on the skin that can vary in shape and size. They can appear anywhere on the body and may result from the body's reaction to specific allergens. Other triggers include infections, stress, extreme temperatures, physical exertion, and certain medications. Acute hives last less than six weeks, while chronic hives persist for over six weeks, sometimes lasting for several years. Despite being uncomfortable and possibly disrupting sleep and daily activities, hives are generally harmless and vanish within 24 hours without leaving any marks.

Sunburn

Sunburn is a skin injury caused by excessive exposure to the sun's ultraviolet (UV) rays or other UV light sources. The skin reddens and becomes painful, and in severe cases, blisters can develop. Other symptoms can include swelling, itching, and peeling skin. Over the long term, repeated sunburns can expedite skin aging and elevate the risk of skin cancer. The best way to protect the skin includes preventing sunburn by seeking shade, donning protective clothing, and applying sunscreen.

Herbal Remedies for the Most Common Skin Conditions

There exist numerous natural remedies that can bolster skin health and aid in managing skin conditions like acne, eczema, psoriasis, and more. These herbs often come with anti-inflammatory, antibacterial, or antioxidant properties.

Acne

Tea Tree Oil (Melaleuca alternifolia): Derived from the Melaleuca alternifolia plant leaves native to Australia, tea tree oil has been employed for hundreds of years as an antimicrobial and antifungal agent. It contains a variety of compounds, including terpinen-4-ol, which is proven to eliminate certain types of bacteria, viruses, and fungi. Terpinen-4-ol also enhances the performance of your white blood cells, contributing to the combat against acne-triggering bacteria.

In relation to acne, the antibacterial characteristics of tea tree oil can aid in tackling Propionibacterium acnes, the bacteria behind follicle inflammation and subsequent acne outbreaks. Furthermore, the oil's anti-inflammatory qualities assist in diminishing the swelling and redness associated with acne, thereby reducing their visibility.

Green Tea (Camellia sinensis): Green tea is abundant in antioxidants known as catechins, which are recognized for their ability to combat inflammation and limit the production of sebum (oil) in the skin. Epigallocatechin gallate (EGCG) is one of the most potent and studied catechins present in green tea, known for its robust antioxidant, anti-inflammatory, and antimicrobial properties.

When used topically, green tea extract can aid in limiting sebum production and curbing acne development. Its anti-inflammatory properties may also help to alleviate the inflammation associated with acne.

Eczema

Chamomile (Matricaria recutita): Often recognized as a soothing ingredient in tea, chamomile also provides impressive benefits for the skin. It's abundant in flavonoids and antioxidants that shield the skin from free radicals, which induce aging.

Chamomile exhibits anti-inflammatory and antimicrobial actions. It can help pacify skin irritations, diminish inflammation, and manage skin conditions like eczema. Its antimicrobial nature can also ward off infection and promote healing, making it valuable in dealing with eczema flare-ups.

Calendula (Calendula officinalis): Calendula encompasses numerous antioxidants, including flavonoids and carotenoids, that aid in skin repair.

Often, Calendula is utilized to calm and moisturize the skin, heal wounds, and alleviate eczema. The plant carries anti-fungal, anti-inflammatory, and antibacterial characteristics that might make it effective in wound healing, pacifying eczema, and easing diaper rash. It's also employed for its wound-healing properties given its ability to boost blood flow and oxygen to the concerned area, assisting the body in generating new tissue and accelerating healing.

Psoriasis

Aloe Vera (Aloe barbadensis miller): The gel-like substance inside its leaves holds various bioactive compounds, including vitamins, antioxidants, and amino acids.

For those grappling with psoriasis, aloe vera can soothe the skin, diminish inflammation and scaling, and enhance the skin's natural healing process. Topical use of aloe vera in the shape of a gel or cream can help hydrate the skin, relieve itchiness, and lower the redness and scaling linked with psoriasis.

Turmeric (Curcuma longa): In relation to psoriasis, curcumin may aid in reducing inflammation and the overproduction of skin cells resulting in psoriasis plaques. Research suggests that topical curcumin application can enhance psoriasis symptoms.

Rosacea

Green Tea (Camellia sinensis): In the case of rosacea, green tea's anti-inflammatory properties can help lessen redness and inflammation. Topical use of green tea extract may help to calm the skin and lower the redness and visible blood vessels related to rosacea.

Licorice (Glycyrrhiza glabra): It encompasses a compound named glycyrrhizin, recognized for its strong anti-inflammatory and immune-boosting properties.

As a topical solution, licorice can help soothe the skin, diminish inflammation, and ease the redness and irritation linked with rosacea. Furthermore, licorice may also aid in enhancing skin hydration and fostering a more even skin tone.

Contact Dermatitis

Witch Hazel (Hamamelis virginiana): Witch hazel, a plant found in North America and parts of Asia, has been recognized for its medicinal attributes for many generations. Its potent anti-inflammatory and astringent characteristics come from the tannins it houses.

In dealing with contact dermatitis, witch hazel can soothe the skin, decrease inflammation, and alleviate itching. Topical usage of witch hazel delivers a refreshing sensation that may assist in calming the discomfort associated with contact dermatitis, lessen inflammation, and deter further irritation or infection.

Herbs for Issues with Hair Loss, Dandruff, and Scalp Conditions

Maintaining the health of hair and scalp is a vital aspect of personal hygiene, and various factors can give rise to conditions like hair loss, dandruff, and other scalp-related issues. Herbal remedies can address these problems, thanks to their advantageous attributes. Let's explore some herbs beneficial for these conditions.

Hair Loss

Rosemary (Rosmarinus officinalis): Rosemary is lauded for its capability to promote hair growth. Using rosemary oil on the scalp can bolster blood circulation, encouraging hair growth and curbing hair loss.

Lavender (Lavandula angustifolia): Lavender oil has demonstrated a capacity to stimulate hair growth by augmenting the number of hair follicles. Its tranquilizing aroma also makes it a favorite choice for relaxation and stress reduction, which can, in turn, assist in averting hair loss triggered by stress.

Dandruff

Tea Tree Oil (Melaleuca alternifolia): The antifungal properties of tea tree oil can help combat the fungus responsible for dandruff. Incorporating a few drops of this oil to your regular shampoo can assist in controlling dandruff.

Neem (Azadirachta indica): Neem, also referred to as Indian lilac, is a medicinal herb that's been employed for thousands of years to remedy various ailments. Neem leaves and oil carry powerful antifungal and antibacterial properties that make them effective in treating dandruff, a common scalp issue.

The antifungal properties of neem help combat the yeast that results in dandruff, and its anti-inflammatory properties can soothe an irritated, itchy scalp. Neem can be employed as an oil or as a rinse, with the leaves steeped in boiling water, cooled, and then used on the scalp and hair.

Scalp Conditions (such as Psoriasis or Dermatitis)

Aloe Vera (Aloe barbadensis miller): Aloe vera's calming properties can help alleviate scalp irritation and inflammation, making it suitable for conditions like psoriasis or dermatitis.

Calendula (Calendula officinalis): Calendula is recognized for its healing, soothing, and anti-inflammatory attributes. It can be applied topically to the scalp to ease irritation and inflammation.

General Scalp Care

Peppermint (Mentha × piperita): Peppermint, a crossbred mint plant, is famous for its invigorating scent. For centuries, it's been employed for its healing benefits, including its capacity to ease digestive problems and soothe headaches.

In the context of hair care, peppermint oil can boost blood circulation to the scalp, which can foster robust hair growth. It also delivers a refreshing, cooling sensation, making it a favored ingredient in hair care products. Some research indicates that peppermint oil might even enhance follicle depth and quantity, leading to denser, fuller hair.

Nettle (Urtica dioica): It's a rich source of vitamins A, C, D, K, and B, and also minerals like iron, potassium, and manganese.

In relation to hair wellness, nettle can help regulate scalp oil production, making it advantageous for both dry and oily scalps. For individuals with oily hair, nettle can aid in reducing excess sebum production, while for those with dry hair, it can assist in moisturization. Nettle can be utilized as a hair rinse by infusing the leaves in boiling water, or it can be applied as an oil directly to the scalp.

Herbal Facial Steam and Herbal Bath

Herbal facial steam is an age-old skincare ritual that entails inhaling steam infused with an array of herbs. It's a straightforward and efficient way to unclog pores, let the skin breathe, and soak up the beneficial attributes of the chosen herbs.

The choice of herbs for a facial steam can be adjusted to meet individual skin requirements. For instance, lavender has soothing properties that can alleviate sensitive or irritated skin, while also delivering a calming aroma that can diminish stress. Chamomile, possessing anti-inflammatory properties, can help mitigate skin redness and irritation, making it a suitable choice for those with skin conditions like rosacea or acne. Rose petals can also be used for their astringent and cooling properties, beneficial for tightening pores and soothing the skin.

To prepare a herbal facial steam, the chosen herbs are infused in boiling water. The individual then leans over the steaming water, with a towel over their head to capture the steam, and inhales deeply. This process usually lasts for around 10-15 minutes, followed by a cold rinse to close the pores and retain the herbal advantages.

Herbal Bath

Herbal baths have been foundational to natural healing and relaxation practices for generations. They can turn a simple bath into a calming, fragrant, and therapeutic session that nurtures the body and soothes the mind.

Different herbs can offer varied benefits in a bath. Calendula, recognized for its soothing properties, can be employed to alleviate irritated or inflamed skin. Lavender, with its tranquilizing scent, can assist in reducing stress and encouraging restful sleep, making it a favored selection for evening baths. Rosemary, with its energizing aroma, can revitalize and refresh the senses, making it an excellent choice for a morning or mid-day bath.

To create a herbal bath, herbs can be wrapped in a cloth or sachet and infused in the bathwater or boiled in water and then added to the bath. It's advised to soak for at least 15-20 minutes to let the body absorb the herbal benefits.

Chapter Ten: Your Own Herbal Garden

Setting up your own herb garden can be an enriching task, both in terms of personal fulfillment and the practical advantages of having a supply of fresh herbs at your disposal. When outlining an herb garden, several elements must be taken into account to assure robust growth and maximum yield. Here are some pivotal considerations:

Locale

Choosing an appropriate location is one of the key facets of nurturing a fruitful herb garden. The correct location can considerably influence the health and output of your herbs. Here are the factors you need to consider:

Sunlight: Sunlight is an essential component for most herbs' growth. They require a generous amount of sunlight to perform photosynthesis effectively, which allows them to grow and generate the flavors and fragrances we appreciate. Ideally, your herb garden should get about 6-8 hours of direct sunlight each day. Nevertheless, if your locale is especially warm, some afternoon shade could be beneficial for your herbs to prevent them from wilting or getting burned.

Soil: Soil is another key determinant for your herb garden. Most herbs favor well-draining soil as water-saturated roots can result in decay and disease. The soil should be abundant in organic matter to deliver the necessary nutrients for your herbs to thrive. However, it should not be overly fertile, as excess nutrients can lead to excessive foliage growth at the expense of essential oils' concentration that gives herbs their distinctive flavors and aromas.

Accessibility: When outlining your herb garden, consider how frequently you'll need to access it for watering, harvesting, and routine upkeep. Ideally, it should be within convenient reach of your home and a water source. Having it close to your kitchen can be particularly useful if you'll be utilizing the herbs for cooking.

Herb Selection

Here's what you should take into account:

Climate: Climate has a significant part in determining which types of herbs you can grow successfully. Some herbs like basil, rosemary, and thyme adore warm and sunny weather, while others like parsley, cilantro, and dill favor cooler conditions. Carry out some research to understand which herbs are best suited to your local climate and consider starting with those for the optimal outcome.

Purpose: The planned use of your herbs is another crucial factor in deciding what to cultivate. If you love to cook and desire fresh herbs at your disposal, consider growing culinary herbs like basil, parsley, rosemary, thyme, and oregano. If you're intrigued by the medicinal properties of herbs, you might select plants like echinacea, lemon balm, calendula, or chamomile. If you're keen on attracting pollinators, consider herbs like lavender, sage, or mint.

Also, think about the flavors and fragrances you relish most and incorporate those in your herb garden.

Planting

Correct plantation is crucial to preparing your herbs for flourishing:

Spacing: Ensuring proper spacing between plants is critical to confirm that each herb gets sufficient room to grow and prosper without competition for sunlight, water, and nutrients. The exact spacing requirements may differ for each herb, so be certain to verify this for each kind of herb you're planting. A general guideline suggests providing 1-2 feet between most herb plants as a good beginning.

Companion Planting: The concept of companion planting implies cultivating certain plants together for mutual advantage. Some herbs can boost each other's growth, improve flavor, and even assist in pest repulsion. For instance, cultivating basil with tomatoes is thought to enrich their flavor and ward off pests. Similarly, planting chives and roses together can help resist black spot, a frequent fungal disease of roses. Always carry out some research or consult a reliable companion planting guide before finalizing your herb garden layout.

Maintenance and Care

Providing appropriate care to your herb garden will help ensure a thriving and abundant harvest. Here are some basic maintenance and care tips:

Watering: Correct watering is one of the keys to a fruitful herb garden. Overwatering is a frequent error when cultivating herbs, as most herbs favor somewhat arid conditions. The guideline is to water thoroughly but occasionally, waiting until the soil is dry to the touch before watering again. The precise frequency will depend on your climate, the time of year, and the specific herbs you are growing.

Weeding: Regular weeding is important to aid your herbs' growth by reducing competition for nutrients, water, and sunlight. Stay vigilant for any unwanted plants, and eliminate them promptly to keep your herb garden in prime condition.

Harvesting: Routine harvesting or pruning stimulates more growth and can assist in keeping your herbs dense and productive. However, when you harvest, never remove more than a third of the plant at a time to avoid causing stress to the plant.

Perennial vs. Annual Herbs

Grasping the difference between perennial and annual herbs is vital when outlining your herb garden.

Perennial herbs are those that regrow every year without needing to be replanted. They include herbs like rosemary, mint, thyme, and oregano. Once established, perennials can be quite resilient and require less upkeep than annuals, but they often need more space to grow and can take longer to reach maturity. Also, some perennial herbs, like mint, can become intrusive if not restricted.

Annual herbs, in contrast, complete their life cycle in a single growing season. This means they sprout, flower, generate seeds, and die within one year. Annual herbs include basil, dill, cilantro, and summer savory. While these herbs need to be replanted each year, they typically grow faster and start producing usable leaves more rapidly than perennials. This makes them an excellent choice if you're seeking a quick harvest.

Starting from Seeds vs. Young Plants

When it comes to initiating your herb garden, you can choose to start from seeds or acquire young plants, often known as 'starts' or 'seedlings,' from a plant nursery.

Starting herbs from seeds can be a gratifying process, and it's often more economical, particularly if you're envisioning a large herb garden. However, it demands more patience and attention. Seeds need the appropriate conditions to sprout, including the correct temperature and moisture levels. Some seeds may also require unique treatment to sprout, such as stratification (exposure to cold) or scarification (scraping or piercing the seed coat).

Conversely, purchasing young plants from a nursery can give you an advantage. These plants are generally several weeks to a few months old and are prepared to be moved into your garden. This can be a quicker and simpler way to initiate your herb garden, especially if you're a novice. However, it can be more costly, and your choice of herbs may be restricted to what's available at the nursery.

Designing and tending an herbal garden can be a satisfying project, furnishing you with an abundance of fresh herbs to utilize in your kitchen or for crafting herbal remedies. With meticulous planning and considerate care, you can build a lush, fruitful garden in your own backyard.

Harvesting, Drying, and Storing Your Herbs

The best moment to harvest herbs is in the morning, precisely after the dew has evaporated but before the day gets hot. This timing is critical as herbs usually have a higher concentration of essential oils during this period. Essential oils are volatile compounds that offer herbs their unique smells and flavors, and they also possess numerous therapeutic properties. In the morning, the plant is fully hydrated, the essential oils are at their highest concentration, and have not yet been degraded or vaporized by the sun's heat. Thus, the aroma and flavor of the herb are preserved at their best.

The prime time to harvest various parts of a plant differs based on what you are aiming to gather. Here is a general guideline:

Leaves: To obtain the greatest concentration of active ingredients, leaves should be harvested before the plant blooms. The plant's energy is most focused in the leaves at this time, making it rich in the compounds you wish to collect.

Flowers: If you are gathering flowers, the ideal time to do so is just as they unfurl. This is when they are at their most vivid, containing maximum levels of essential oils and medicinal compounds.

Roots: For root harvest, autumn is the best season, especially after the plant's foliage has started to fade. At this stage, the plant's energy moves downwards to the roots for winter storage, resulting in a concentration of active constituents in the roots.

Seeds: Seeds should be gathered when they are mature and dry on the plant. This indicates that the seeds have reached their peak nutritional or medicinal value.

It's vital to harvest herbs in a way that allows the plant to recover and continue growing. The general rule of thumb is not to remove more than a third of the plant at one time. This leaves enough foliage to allow the plant to photosynthesize and regenerate. Overharvesting can stress the plant and may lead to stunted growth or even death.

Furthermore, using clean, sharp tools for harvesting is highly advised. Clean tools prevent the spread of disease among plants, while sharp tools help ensure clean cuts. A clean cut is less likely to cause damage to the plant, aiding in faster recovery and preventing the entry of diseases. It's also beneficial for the harvested parts as they are less likely to wilt or degrade quickly if the cuts are clean and precise.

Drying

Once you've gathered your herbs, wash them with care and pat dry. Several techniques can be employed to dry herbs:

Air-Drying: This straightforward, age-old practice of preserving herbs works well for a variety of types. To air-dry herbs, group them in a loose bunch and hang them inverted in a space that's warm, dry, and shadowy, with adequate airflow to ward off mold. The upside-down position facilitates the essential oils' migration from the stems to the leaves. The duration of this process might range from 1 to 2 weeks, contingent on the specific herbs and the environmental conditions.

This method, however, doesn't work well for herbs with high moisture content like basil, chives, or mint, as they might become moldy before they are thoroughly dried.

Oven-Drying: If you're looking to dry your herbs more rapidly, oven-drying presents a handy alternative. To oven-dry herbs, arrange them in a single layer on a baking sheet and place them in an oven set to the lowest possible heat setting. For optimal air circulation, the oven door should be left slightly open. It's crucial to periodically monitor the herbs to avoid them from scorching or turning brown, which would signal the loss of essential oils.

This approach can be swifter than air-drying, but it calls for vigilant oversight to avoid the herbs from overheating, which can result in loss of taste and medicinal attributes.

Using a Dehydrator: A food dehydrator serves as an efficient apparatus for drying herbs, particularly if you have a large quantity. Dehydrators are engineered to extract moisture from food at a controlled temperature, thereby preserving the flavor and nutritional profile of the herbs.

To dry herbs in a dehydrator, all you need to do is lay the herbs out on the provided trays and adhere to the guidelines associated with your specific model. Bear in mind that different herbs might necessitate varying drying times and temperatures.

Storing

Once your herbs have fully dried, it's crucial to ensure they're stowed in a way that retains their therapeutic properties:

Preserving Dried Herbs in Sealed Containers: It's of utmost importance to keep your herbs in an appropriate container after they have completely dried to enhance their longevity and safeguard their taste and strength. Ideal containers for preserving dried herbs are those that are sealed tight, such as glass jars. Containers that are sealed restrict the entry of moisture and air, averting the possibility of your herbs becoming moldy or losing their strength. To avoid the degradation of your herbs from sunlight, leading to loss of color, flavor, and medicinal value, keep these containers away from direct light. A cool, shaded spot like a pantry or cupboard serves as the perfect place.

Tagging the Jars: It's wise to mark each jar with the herb's name and the date it was stored. This may appear unessential initially, especially if you feel you can distinguish each herb by its look or fragrance. Nonetheless, dried herbs can end up looking surprisingly alike, and their scent can fade as time passes. Marking the date of storage helps you monitor their age, letting you know when they should be replaced.

Best Before of Dried Herbs: Despite the ability of dried herbs to be kept for an extended period, they deliver the best results if used within a year. Gradually, the potency of even the most meticulously stored herbs will wane. A reliable sign that your dried herbs are still suitable for use is if they maintain their color and fragrance. If the hue has significantly faded or the scent is faint or missing, it's probable that the herbs have lost their strength and it might be time to replenish them.

Maintaining the Herbs Intact: One strategy to ensure your herbs stay potent for as long as feasible is to keep them whole until the time you're ready to utilize them. When herbs are ground or broken down, a larger surface area is exposed to air, light, and warmth, which can accelerate the depletion of the essential oils that lend herbs their unique flavor and medicinal attributes. By preserving them intact, you're safeguarding these essential oils and confirming that your herbs are as powerful as they can be when you put them to use.

Tips for Gardening Practices

Constructing a therapeutic herb garden can provide an abundant source of curative flora and also contribute positively to our Earth's health if executed in a sustainable manner. Here are the common horticultural methodologies for growing medicinal herbs:

Conservation of Water: One of the simplest strategies to economize water is by employing drip watering systems or absorption hoses, which supply water straight to the root system of the plants, limiting evaporation. Storing rainwater in barrels presents another effective approach to utilize natural resources. Additionally, mulching your plants aids in moisture retention and lessens the need for frequent watering.

Natural Methods: Refrain from utilizing synthetic fertilizers and insecticides. Instead, choose natural fertilizers such as compost, vermicast, or fish by-products. Pests can be managed naturally by promoting the presence of beneficial insects, rotating crops, and applying homemade organic sprays.

Recycling Organic Waste: Recycling organic waste materials like kitchen leftovers, lawn trimmings, and fallen leaves creates a fertile environment for your garden. It's an efficient method to reuse plant materials and reduce the volume of waste headed for the landfill. Furthermore, it boosts soil fertility and cultivates healthier plants.

Maintaining Soil Quality: A healthy soil serves as the cornerstone of a prosperous garden. Regularly enrich your soil with organic matter to enhance its structure and nutrient content. Implement crop rotation and cover cropping to sustain soil fertility and prevent diseases.

Indigenous Plants: Cultivating indigenous plants aids in preserving regional biodiversity. These plants are adjusted to the local climate and soil conditions, hence require less maintenance. They also serve as habitats for local wildlife.

Mindful Harvesting: Steer clear of excessive harvesting, which can put plants under stress and decrease their lifespan. As a general guideline, refrain from taking more than a third of the plant at a time, and provide the plant plenty of recovery time before the subsequent harvest. Certain plants, like perennial roots, should only be harvested every few years.

Seed Preservation and Plant Multiplication: By preserving seeds and multiplying plants, you can preserve plant diversity, adapt plants to your local conditions, and lessen the necessity to purchase new plants each year.

Ecological Design: Arrange your garden to minimize its environmental footprint. This might involve strategic positioning of plants to maximize sunlight exposure, creating wind barriers to shield delicate plants, or even establishing a rain garden to manage stormwater runoff.

Bonus Chapter: Global Herbal Traditions

Herbal therapeutics has firmly anchored itself in the customs of diverse cultures worldwide.

Ayurveda, the term meaning "life's knowledge," is a comprehensive medicinal system with roots in India, dating back more than three millennia. It categorizes individuals into three distinct doshas (Vata, Pitta, Kapha), each with unique dietary and herbal guidelines. Ayurvedic herbs like Ashwagandha, Turmeric, and Tulsi are frequently employed for their restorative attributes.

Traditional Chinese Medicine, with its own rich history spanning thousands of years, uses herbal concoctions to achieve equilibrium between the body's yin and yang. TCM incorporates an extensive materia medica, encompassing herbs like Ginseng, Astragalus, and Ginkgo Biloba.

Western Herbalism finds its lineage in Greek and Roman traditions, but it also borrows extensively from Native American herbal insights. It interprets herbs through the prism of four "humors" or "temperaments" and employs herbs like Echinacea, Valerian, and St. John's Wort.

Unani is a medicinal system originating from Greco-Arabic traditions, with a focus on the four humors (blood, phlegm, yellow bile, and black bile). Plant-based remedies in Unani medicine incorporate Senna, Fenugreek, and Licorice.

African traditional medicine exhibits variations across different regions and tribes. It leans heavily on the knowledge of regional medicinal plants handed down through generations. African medicinal flora includes the African potato, Devil's claw, and Rooibos.

In the Amazon rainforest, native tribes have cultivated extensive expertise regarding the region's abundant botanical treasures. Medicinal plants from the Amazon encompass Ayahuasca, Cat's Claw, and Pau d'Arco.

Australian Aboriginal people have utilized local flora for healing for several millennia. Notable examples include Tea Tree, Eucalyptus, and Kakadu Plum.

These traditions underscore the point that plants have consistently acted as mankind's allies and healers across time and cultures, and they persist in playing a vital role in our shared health and wellness. As we progress, it's imperative to preserve this timeless knowledge and ensure its passage to subsequent generations.

Ayurveda - The Indian System of Herbal Medicine

Ayurveda, directly translating to "the knowledge of existence," is an age-old medicinal framework from India, with a history stretching over 5000 years. Its fundamental purpose is to impart wisdom regarding the preservation of wellbeing, along with managing ailments through harmony among body, mind, and spirit.

The bedrock of Ayurveda lies in the philosophy of five rudimentary elements or Pancha Mahabhutas: Space (Akasha), Air (Vayu), Fire (Agni), Water (Jala), and Earth (Prithvi).

Doshas: As per Ayurveda, these five constituents intermingle within the human body in varying proportions to give rise to three vital forces or biological energies, called doshas: Vata (Space and Air), Pitta (Fire and Water), and Kapha (Water and Earth).

Vata: The power of movement, it commands all physical motions and actions within our bodies, such as respiration, blinking, blood flow, muscular and tissue movement, along with cardiac operations.

Pitta: The power governing digestion and metabolism, it oversees all transformative actions including digestion, absorption, assimilation, nutrition, thermoregulation, skin pigmentation, and intellect.

Kapha: The force of lubrication and structure, it ensures growth, lends mass to our bodies, lubricates joints, and provides a cooling effect to balance out Pitta's heat.

Distinct Dosha Combinations: It is believed that each individual possesses a distinctive mix of these three doshas, decided at the instant of conception, referred to as their Prakriti or constitutional make-up. This Prakriti outlines a person's physical, mental, and emotional traits.

Health and Disease: In the Ayurvedic view, health represents a state where doshas are balanced, while disease arises from their imbalance. Various factors such as stress, unhealthy food habits, changes in weather, and incorrect lifestyle can trigger imbalance.

Role of Herbs in Ayurveda

In the context of Ayurveda, herbs are instrumental in upholding and restoring the equilibrium of the doshas. They are perceived as powerful therapeutic agents carrying different tastes, energies, post-digestive effects, and particular actions that influence the doshas.

Powerful Therapeutic Instruments: Herbs are often amalgamated in Ayurvedic concoctions in line with a distinct herbal science named "Synergy". This principle proposes that herbs, when combined, amplify each other's curative effects and reduce potential side effects. For instance, in a conventional Ayurvedic compound named Triphala, three fruits (Amalaki, Haritaki, and Bibhitaki) are mixed, each impacting different doshas, thus creating a balanced and potent formulation.

Influence of Various Factors: The selection of herbs and their usage in Ayurveda is influenced by several aspects. These include the individual's constitution (Prakriti), the dominant dosha that is out of balance (Vikriti), the disease's nature and phase, the individual's age and strength, the prevailing season, and other environmental factors.

Herbs and Dosha Harmonizing: For instance, if an individual's Vata dosha is unbalanced, herbs with sweet, sour, and salty tastes that are warm, heavy, and oily might be chosen to counterbalance the light, dry, cold, and rough characteristics of Vata. Conversely, if an individual's Pitta dosha is high, cooling, dry, and light herbs with sweet, bitter, and astringent tastes may be deployed.

Ayurvedic Diets and Lifestyles

In Ayurvedic philosophy, the significance of therapeutic substances extends beyond medicines. The approach to eating and daily regimen are also considered pivotal for ensuring vitality and handling ailments. These elements are regarded as primary protective measures against diseases and crucial constituents of the healing process.

Diet: The Ayurvedic approach to nourishment promotes physical vitality and equilibrium among the doshas. The focus is on the consumption of fresh, seasonal, and locally sourced produce, prepared with suitable herbs and spices. Ayurveda proposes that each repast should feature all six flavors - sweet, sour, salty, bitter, pungent, and astringent, to appease all senses and encourage balanced nutrition. The selection of foods is also customized according to the individual's prevailing dosha and the existing season.

A salubrious way of living is also greatly accentuated in Ayurveda, for the advancement of holistic health. This encompasses:

Appropriate Sleep: Sufficient, high-quality sleep is deemed crucial in Ayurveda, on par with a balanced diet for preserving health. The body engages in critical restoration and rejuvenation processes during sleep.

Physical Exertion: Regular physical exercise, particularly yoga, is strongly advised in Ayurveda. Yoga not only sustains bodily flexibility and vitality but also fosters mental lucidity and mitigates stress.

Meditation: Another key component of the Ayurvedic lifestyle is meditation. Consistent meditation practice can alleviate stress, enhance mental clarity, boost concentration, and uplift overall wellbeing.

Routines Tied to Daily and Seasonal Cycles: Ayurveda advocates the observance of specific daily (Dinacharya) and seasonal (Ritucharya) routines to synchronize the body's rhythm with the natural cycles of the sun, the moon, and the changing seasons. These regimens may involve rising early, partaking in purifying practices, eating at suitable intervals, and modifying routines and diet to correspond with the shifting seasons.

The Ayurvedic framework is an exhaustive and integrative approach to health that doesn't merely concentrate on treating symptoms but also seeks to confront the fundamental cause of the disease. It underscores personalized treatment, recognizing that each individual possesses a unique constitution and health state.

An Ancient Practice of Traditional Chinese Medicine

Traditional Chinese Medicine is an all-encompassing health system that has matured and evolved for over two millennia. This system encompasses various therapeutic methods, including acupuncture, massage, dietary practices, and notably, the use of medicinal herbs, for diagnosing and managing health issues.

At the foundation of TCM lies the notion of Qi (voiced as 'chee'), or the vital life force. According to TCM, wellness is realized when Qi in the body is balanced and flows without obstruction. Conversely, disease is seen as a consequence of imbalances or blockages of Qi.

Moreover, the guiding principle of Yin-Yang, the two counteractive yet synergistic forces that govern the cosmos and all life within it, is intrinsic to TCM. Harmonizing these forces within the body is fundamental for preserving health.

In TCM, herbal therapies are pivotal in restoring and maintaining the balance of Qi and Yin-Yang within the body. TCM herbology encompasses a wide range of plants, animal products, and minerals, each with distinctive characteristics and effects. Most commonly, herbs are amalgamated into intricate formulas devised to address specific patterns of imbalance. Frequently utilized herbs include Ginseng, Astragalus, Dong Quai, Licorice.

The Integrative Approach

Similar to Ayurveda, TCM adopts a holistic outlook, perceiving the body as a linked system rather than segregated parts. It considers the entirety of an individual's health, encompassing physical, emotional, mental, and environmental elements.

Equilibrium and Unity: Fundamental to TCM philosophy is the concept of equilibrium and unity. An individual's health is understood to be regulated by the balance of Yin and Yang, two contrasting yet complementary forces. Additionally, TCM subscribes to the concept of Qi (voiced as "chee"), a vital energy or life force that circulates within the body via a system of channels known as meridians. Disease is perceived as a result of imbalances in Yin and Yang or obstructions in the Qi flow.

Interrelation with the Environment: TCM also underscores the interdependence of humans and their surroundings. It suggests that external factors such as weather and seasonal transitions can profoundly influence an individual's health and wellness. TCM aims to synchronize the body's rhythms with the natural ebbs and flows of the environment to encourage wellness.

Diet and Lifestyle: Analogous to Ayurveda, TCM strongly accentuates the significance of dietary and lifestyle adaptations. TCM dietary guidelines advocate eating in harmony with the seasons, balancing the five tastes (sweet, sour, bitter, salty, and spicy), and consuming foods that fortify the body's constitution or help balance the disrupted energies.

TCM practitioners take into account the patient's overall constitution, symptoms, and the nature of their illness before devising a personalized treatment plan. The plan typically integrates dietary alterations, lifestyle changes, acupuncture, herbal treatments, Tai Chi, Qigong, and other therapies.

Western Herbalism - Roots and Modern Practices

The herbal knowledge of Europe and North America converges in Western Herbalism, which represents a fusion of ancient medicinal wisdom from the two continents. This system has matured over centuries, incorporating elements from the healing methods of Native Americans, the humoral theory of the Greeks, and modern insights into plant chemistry and physiology.

The origins of Western Herbalism can be traced to the times of the ancient Greeks and Romans, but it also incorporates significant elements from Egyptian and Arabian medicine. Numerous traditional herb usage that originated in the Middle Ages have been passed down and remain in use to this day.

In the Americas, the indigenous populations' expansive knowledge of herbs significantly enriched Western Herbalism. Native American tribes possessed extensive understanding of the flora in their local habitats and used these for a broad spectrum of health conditions.

Principles

In contrast to traditional health systems like Ayurveda or Traditional Chinese Medicine, Western Herbalism does not hinge on a single defining theory or philosophy. Instead, it favors a more practical and varied approach rooted in observation, hands-on experience, and experimentation.

Flora: Western Herbalism regards each plant as possessing a unique mix of medicinal attributes. This viewpoint echoes the tradition of the "Doctrine of Signatures", an ancient philosophy that proposed that herbs resembling various body parts could be employed to treat ailments of those body parts.

Health and Imbalance: In a manner similar to other traditional systems, Western Herbalism sees disease as a signal of an overall body imbalance rather than an isolated incident. Its goal is to uncover the root causes of illness and to restore the body's natural balance.

Evidence-based Approach: Western Herbalism adopts an evidence-based method where knowledge about the medicinal attributes of herbs has been amassed over centuries via practical use and observation. This wealth of information has been passed down through generations and is a critical aspect of the Western herbal tradition.

Modern Practices in Western Herbalism

The practice of Western Herbalism has undergone significant changes with the advent of modern science and technology.

Integration with Scientific Research: Today's Western Herbalists frequently intersect with scientific research. They aim to comprehend the biochemical constituents of herbs, and how these individual elements interact with the human body. Modern technology has facilitated the isolation and examination of active compounds in herbs, providing a scientific foundation for understanding their therapeutic impacts.

Amalgamation of Tradition and Modern Science: Despite the infusion of scientific research, modern Western Herbalism continues to place high value on the wisdom and knowledge derived from traditional herb usage. It represents a mix of tradition and science, where contemporary scientific discoveries are employed to corroborate and enhance traditional herbal therapies.

Diverse Modes of Practice: Western Herbalism in the present day is practiced in a wide variety of forms. These range from professional clinical herbalists who work with clients much like other healthcare providers, to home herbalists who cultivate, gather, and utilize herbs for the everyday health needs of their families.

Holistic View: Like other herbal traditions, Western Herbalism approaches health from a holistic perspective. It takes into account the entire person, their surroundings, diet, and lifestyle when devising a treatment plan. The goal is not merely to relieve symptoms but to restore balance and bolster the body's innate healing capacity.

The Future of Herbal Medicine - Trends and Possibilities

Looking forward, it's evident that botanical remedies will remain a crucial component in the sphere of global health. With the emergence of advanced scientific methodologies and a revived enthusiasm for natural healing techniques, the potential for the growth of herbal medicine is increasing at a rapid pace.

Symbiosis with Contemporary Medicine

The idea of melding herbal medicine with contemporary medical practices is gaining traction. This combined method, often dubbed as integrative or complementary medicine, is acquiring acceptance among medical professionals and patients alike. Here's a glimpse into how this unification is evolving:

All-encompassing Treatment: Marrying herbal medicine with modern medicine facilitates an all-encompassing therapeutic approach. While modern medicine is often efficient in managing symptoms and acute conditions, herbal medicine can augment this by aiding in tackling underlying disparities and fostering overall wellbeing.

Tailored Care: Integrative medicine acknowledges the individual variances among patients and strives to deliver personalized care. By taking into account the patient's unique health condition, lifestyle, and preferences, healthcare practitioners can combine the finest elements from both worlds to devise a treatment regimen that fits the individual patient.

Proactive Healthcare: Herbal medicine can also play a role in proactive healthcare. Numerous herbs are renowned for their immune-enhancing, stress-alleviating, and other health-boosting properties. When fused with modern medicine, these properties can contribute to the overall proactive health strategy.

Investigation and Innovation

Herbal medicine is indeed undergoing a scientific renaissance, with advanced technologies being leveraged to investigate medicinal plants and develop more potent herbal products.

Sophisticated Methods: Methods such as genetic sequencing and metabolomics are being utilized to probe the curative potential of plants at the molecular level. Genetic sequencing aids in identifying medicinal plants and examining their evolutionary traits, while metabolomics is employed to identify and quantify the metabolic compounds present in these plants.

Unveiling of New Compounds: The employment of these sophisticated techniques could result in the unveiling of new medicinal compounds. These newly unveiled compounds could introduce new therapeutic uses or could be utilized to devise new drugs for existing health conditions.

Product Enhancement: The insights gleaned from such research are also being employed to enhance herbal products. For instance, understanding the precise composition of a plant can aid in standardizing herbal extracts, ensuring their efficacy and safety.

Personalized Herbal Medicine

The ascension of personalized medicine is also leaving its mark on the domain of herbal medicine.

Genomic Analysis: Genomic analysis can aid in discerning an individual's susceptibility to certain ailments and their potential response to specific herbs. This data can direct the choice of botanical remedies, resulting in a more customized and potentially efficacious treatment.

Sophisticated Diagnostics: Sophisticated diagnostic tools can afford a more intricate understanding of a person's health condition. By amalgamating this with knowledge of herbal medicine, practitioners can fine-tune treatment strategies to cater to the specific requirements of each individual.

Customized Therapeutic Plans: The future trajectory of herbal medicine likely encompasses more customized therapeutic plans. These plans would consider a person's unique genetic profile, health condition, lifestyle, and preferences, leading to a more personalized and holistic approach to healthcare.

Preservation and Sustainability

The escalating demand for herbal products calls for a crucial emphasis on preservation and sustainability. This necessity emerges from several concerns:

Excessive Harvesting: Excessive harvesting poses a significant menace to numerous medicinal plant species. With the growing popularity of herbal medicine, many wild plant populations are being exploited at unsustainable rates, which may lead to their depletion or extinction.

Global Warming: Global warming presents another hurdle, as shifts in temperature, rainfall patterns, and increased occurrence of severe weather events can adversely impact the natural habitats of these plants.

Sustainable Farming: To combat these threats, strides are being taken towards sustainable farming practices. This comprises practices like organic agriculture, agroforestry, and harvesting protocols that ensure the plants can regenerate.

Conservation Initiatives: The conservation of medicinal plants is essential to safeguard these resources for forthcoming generations. This incorporates strategies like seed banking, in-situ (on-site) and ex-situ (off-site) conservation, and policies to protect wild populations and their habitats.

Education and Regulation

With herbal medicine moving more into the limelight, there's a growing demand for more rigorous oversight and enlightenment:

Oversight: More stringent regulatory measures are essential to guarantee the quality, safety, and effectiveness of herbal products. This incorporates rigorous quality control norms, accurate product labeling, and scrutiny of product claims.

Enlightenment: Parallel in importance is the necessity to illuminate both practitioners and the public regarding the safe and effective utilization of herbal medicine. This entails training for healthcare providers in herbal medicine, and public education initiatives to inform users about safe usage, possible interactions, and how to select high-quality products.

Digital Innovation in Herbal Medicine

Digital innovation is ushering in thrilling developments in the realm of herbal medicine:

Remote Consultations: Telemedicine is enabling individuals to seek advice from professional herbalists from the convenience of their own homes. This is especially advantageous for those in isolated locations or with mobility constraints.

Plant Identification Apps: Applications are being designed that can assist in identifying medicinal plants, offer information about their applications, and even instruct users on how to gather and prepare them.

AI-Powered Tools: Looking forward, we can anticipate further advancements like AI-powered tools that can scrutinize personal health data and customize herbal remedy suggestions to individual needs.

Internet-Based Education Platforms: Digital technology is also transforming education in herbal medicine. Online courses, webinars, and resources permit anyone with an internet connection to gain knowledge about herbs, their applications, and their benefits.

Afterword

My hope is that this guide has ignited a spark within you and piqued your interest in the practice of harnessing plant-derived solutions to augment wellness and address health challenges. It's a realm that merges ancestral wisdom with modern scientific insights, offering us an alternate and supplementary route to sustain and regain our health.

Plant-based remedies, though rooted in antiquity, are far from being mere historical artifacts. Today, our relationship with nature can often be tense, and these remedies act as a conduit, linking us to the earth's inherent healing powers. They serve as a reminder that health and recovery are within our grasp, often just a stone's throw away, waiting to be unearthed and harnessed.

Looking towards the future, the prospects for the field of herbal medicine are enormous. With an ever-expanding volume of research substantiating its advantages, and an escalating awareness of the need for sustainable and attainable health solutions, the future of herbal medicine seems bright.

Thank you for investing your time in reading my book. To your health and wellbeing, and may your journey be perpetually verdant!